THINKING MAN Diet

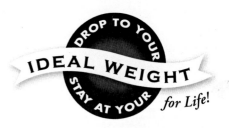

BOBB BIEHL

Published by Aylen Publishing
www.BobbBiehl.com

Subject Heading: 1. Diet and Weight 2. Self-Help

ISBN 978-0-98577080-8

THINKING MAN Diet

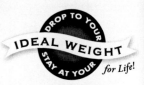

DROP TO YOUR
IDEAL WEIGHT
STAY AT YOUR *for Life!*

There are three very different kinds of diets ...

	WEIGHT LOSS	PHYSICAL FITNESS	NUTRITION
What do you actually want from this book?	Look like James Bond /007 in a tux ... business suit ... dress casual?	Look like Mr. Universe in a Speedo?	Look like Dr. Healthy?
Realistically, what are you willing to do at this point in your life?	**THINK** Think about your weight ... think differently about food ... and, simply eat less of what you enjoy eating ...	**EXERCISE** Exercise an hour a day ... running, swimming, weights, treadmill ... eat different foods, take expensive supplements ...	**CHANGE** Change what you eat ... to far healthier foods, eating new foods, take diet supplements; stop eating foods you really enjoy, count calories ...
How public are you willing to be with your diet at the moment?	**IN-VISIBLE** No one sees, notices, comments ... until you have lost weight!	**VERY-VISIBLE** Everyone knows you have joined a health club ... everyone at the club or in the neighborhood watches you working out, swigging diet drinks, taking your pills!	**VERY-VISIBLE** Everyone sees you eating foods you never have before ... everyone sees and comments on what you are eating, taking and drinking!
What book would be most likely read ... TODAY?	**THINKING MAN DIET** *DROP to YOUR "IDEAL WEIGHT"* *STAY at YOUR "IDEAL WEIGHT"*	**NO MEAT ATHLETE** *Run on Plants and Discover Your Fittest, Fastest, Happiest Self*	**THAT'S WHY WE DON'T EAT ANIMALS:** *A Book About Vegans, Vegetarians, and All Living Things*
What would you like your friend to say?	You've lost weight! You look great!	You've been working out! You look great!	Are you a Vegan? So am I!

	WEIGHT LOSS	PHYSICAL FITNESS	NUTRITION
At this point in your life which <u>plan</u> do you need?	A step-by-step plan to get to my "IDEAL WEIGHT" and stay there for life.	A step-by-step plan to get in peek physical shape.	A step-by-step plan to count carbs, take supplements, balance types of food, and, not eat certain foods.
Realistically, if you will only start one diet which will it be?	**WEIGHT LOSS DIET** The **THINKING MAN Diet** has been designed for you!	**PHYSICAL FITNESS DIET** Read **THINKING MAN Diet** as a supplement to your exercise regimen.	**NUTRITION DIET** Read **THINKNG MAN Diet** as a supplement to your nutritional program.

Obviously, we would like to have all three. Realistically, trying all three at once is overwhelming to most people. Most thinking men think about developing most projects in phases. What would be your phase preference?

Weight loss first?

Physical fitness first?

Nutrition first?

THINK ABOUT IT:

A man CAN NOT realistically achieve physical fitness or true health ... when he is way over weight!

Logically, when you get to your "IDEAL WEIGHT" you can focus on PHYSICAL FITNESS AND NUTRITION, if you like.

THE THINKING MAN Diet IS <u>FOCUSED</u> ON WEIGHT LOSS ...

> NOT focused on the latest in running or body building techniques
>
> NOT focused on which foods to eat and not eat / supplements to take
>
> IT IS FOCUSED ON **WEIGHT LOSS!**

If, your real agenda is to:

> DROP to YOUR "IDEAL WEIGHT"
> STAY at YOUR "IDEAL WEIGHT"

Read on!

SATISFIED THINKER

On the THINKING MAN DIET I've now lost over 30 pounds I'm ready for an exercise program that will help me continue on the path to my ideal weight and improve my fitness. And, along with the THINKING MAN DIET I've found I enjoy eating healthier as well. Thank you! — T

At Your

"IDEAL WEIGHT"

You will not hear

(Or, need to think of yourself as ...)

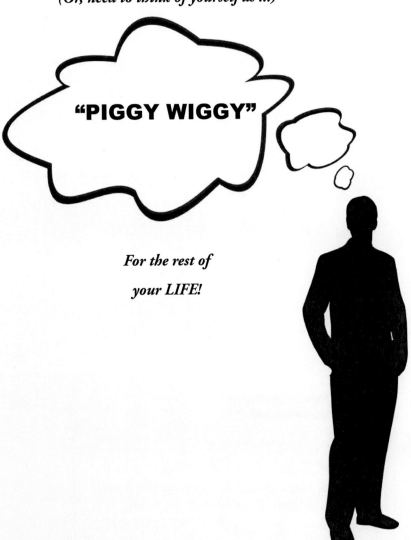

"PIGGY WIGGY"

For the rest of

your LIFE!

CONTENTS

A PERSONAL NOTE

INTRODUCING — A new way of thinking!

CHAPTER 1   UNDERSTANDING — *why "crash diets" work at first, but don't last!*

CHAPTER 2   DECIDING — *Your "IDEAL WEIGHT"*

CHAPTER 3   THINKING — *for yourself!*

CHAPTER 4   WEIGHING — *yourself every morning!*

CHAPTER 5   SAVORING — *every bite!*

CHAPTER 6   EATING AND DRINKING — *whatever you want, just less of it!*

CHAPTER 7   UNLEARNING — *"clean up your plate"!*

CHAPTER 8   KEEPING — *your new thinking a secret!*

CHAPTER 9   WATCHING — *your self image turn far more positive!*

CHAPTER 10   STARTING — *today step-by-step toward your "IDEAL WEIGHT"!*

A PERSONAL NOTE

Over a period of about 8 months (telling no one I was on a diet) I dropped from 203 pounds to 160 pounds!
And, have easily and consistently kept the weight off!

Many friends asked me, *"How did you TAKE IT OFF? ... how do you KEEP IT OFF?"* I decided to carefully analyze and write down how I actually did it.

This book explains how I actually got to my "IDEAL WEIGHT" and, details the "THIN THOUGHTS" helping me stay at my "IDEAL WEIGHT" month after month.

I had zero idea of writing a book on this subject ...
>   I'M NOT A CRASH DIET-IST,
>   I'M NOT A DIET EXPERT,
>   I'M NOT A DOCTOR,
>   I'M NOT A NUTRITIONIST,
>   I'M NOT A PHARMACIST,
>   I'M NOT A PHYSICAL THERAPIST,

Honestly, I'm not even perfect in executing 100% of the "THIN THOUGHTS" in this book 100% of the time!

I'm just A REALIST who figured out a profoundly simple combination of "THIN THOUGHTS", which worked for me. **I do not mean in any way to "degrade" any of the approaches below ... they work for many ... these approaches just do not appeal to me!**

The THINKING MAN Diet has:

- No embarrassing support group weekly ("weigh in") ... with a group of obese "temporary friends"

- No grueling painful weight loss exercises / workouts. Exercise is great – but, not required on the THINKING MAN Diet

- No potentially harmful diet pills

- No expensive frozen / dried / powdered "skinny tasting" foods to buy

- No time consuming weight loss camp

- No unhealthy "crash diet" – Knowing at the end ... you will reward yourself with a huge helping of what you have wanted all along!

- NO complex counting or charts to keep

- NO expensive health club to join

IN TOTAL SECRET

I went from the most I had *ever* weighed to my "IDEAL WEIGHT"

and

kept off the embarrassing weight ... with 100% confidence I can "STAY at MY "IDEAL WEIGHT" " for the rest of my life.

I did it simply by *THINKING* about eating and food differently than I have in the past.

I didn't start out with all of the "THIN THOUGHTS" in this book! I started out with just a deep commitment to get to my "IDEAL WEIGHT"! This book, and the "THIN THOUGHTS" in it are a real life, practical, easy to use (and keep a total secret) ... by-product!

Remember, this entire book is just trying to answer 2 questions,

- *How did you Drop to your IDEAL WEIGHT?*

    and,

- *How do you stay at your IDEAL WEIGHT?*

I sincerely hope you can benefit from the 'THINKING MAN Diet" as much as I HAVE ... and, AM!

Bobb
BIEHL

Bobb Biehl
Executive Mentor
Leading, Managing, Living

INTRODUCING – *A new way of thinking*

THINKING – *about eating and food with profoundly simple logic*

Thinking your way ... to your "IDEAL WEIGHT" ... using the THINKING MAN Diet is profoundly simple ... not complex ... it just works!

Here is the most basic logic of the THINKING MAN Diet:

You learn wise ways of:

- Eating what you want to eat ... JUST LESS OF IT!

- Dropping to your "IDEAL WEIGHT"

- Staying under your new "NEVER GO OVER WEIGHT"

- Remembering a series of "THIN THOUGHTS" which become your "NEW NORMAL"

- Keeping your new way of thinking about food and eating (diet) INVISIBLE TO FRIENDS.

"

Bottom line, the THINKING MAN Diet has had a positive impact. Made me stop and think about food and eating, but the important part is that your book taught me HOW to THINK about food and eating.

I was motivated and impacted by...

> *Thinking about food and eating for the first time really.*
>
> *Thinking about how I was eating.*
>
> *Thinking about savoring it.*
>
> *Thinking about going slower.*
>
> *Thinking about eating less of it, leaving just a bit of everything.*

These five "think" items above have played a key role in my dropping 15 to 20 pounds in the past couple of months. Something is working!

Other parts of your book will help others who have been trying diets or are concerned with what others think or see. Not biggies for me. For me ... THINKING internally about the HOW TO THINK about food and eating, was a big hit for me! — C.

PS As a man thinks in his heart, so is he. Proverbs 23:7

"

WARNING —
Starting the THINKING MAN Diet is not for you, if ...

- You have physical problems contributing to your weight issues – or, are at all concerned any diet may cause you problems ... SEE A DOCTOR!

- Your emotional needs make your eating decisions (The THINKING MAN Diet assumes you are emotionally very healthy)

- You are currently under a tremendous amount of stress, or in a major transition. Frankly, now may not the right time to start anything new!

- You eat only candy bars and "junk food" ...
  this diet assumes you eat basically healthy foods ...
  just far too much of them. It should be obvious to everyone – if you eat more vegetables and fruits ... less pastries, fried foods, and sugar ... it helps even more!

- You have tried every diet under the sun ... and, nothing works – to help you:

  > Drop to your IDEAL WEIGHT
  > Stay at your IDEAL WEIGHT

  Likely this won't be the "magic formula" for you either.
  If you are unable to commit to a diet... saying you will do it and then cheating... this is not the diet for you.
  To have the THINKING MAN Diet work you need to be committed. If you don't follow it ... it won't work ... it is not a "magic formula"!

- You have "made up your mind" this diet will work for you (for whatever reason) ...
  chances are very good ... IT WON'T!

IF YOU ARE A BINGE-EATER … you are encouraged to seek professional help. Binge-eating is an issue which is beyond the scope of the THINKING MAN Diet.

BINGE EATING
From Wikipedia, the free encyclopedia

Binge eating is a pattern of disordered eating which consists of episodes of uncontrollable eating. It is sometimes as a symptom of binge eating disorder or compulsive overeating disorder. During such binges, a person rapidly consumes an excessive amount of food. Most people who have eating binges try to hide this behavior from others, and often feel ashamed about being overweight or depressed about their overeating. Although people who do not have any eating disorder may occasionally experience episodes of overeating, frequent binge eating is often a symptom of an eating disorder. About one in five young women report that they have had binge-eating symptoms, according to the National Institute of Mental Health. Men account for about 40% of binge-eating disorder symptoms.
Binge-eating disorder, as the name implies, is characterized by uncontrollable, excessive eating, followed by feelings of shame and guilt. Unlike those with bulimia, those with binge-eating disorder symptoms typically do not purge their food. However, many who have bulimia also have binge-eating disorder.
Binge-eaters may use food to fill an emotional void by overeating to cope with life's challenges and with their emotional insecurities. In reality, their overeating causes guilt, shame and disgust. Frequently, they are overweight and typically suffer from low self-esteem. Binge eating is very common mostly with teenagers.

READING – QUICKLY

No man wants to spend the rest of his life reading a book about a diet. This is a "quick read" book which gets to the heart of subjects and quickly moves on!

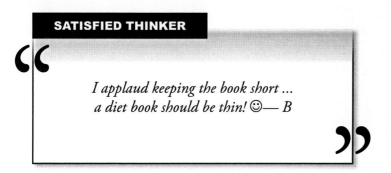

SATISFIED THINKER

I applaud keeping the book short ... a diet book should be thin! ☺— B

HOW I ACTUALLY FEEL ABOUT:
THINKING MAN Diet

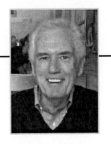

For over 60 years I have felt OVERWEIGHT ... NEVER
to the point of being obese ... but, always overweight.
And, I never ENJOYED IT FOR ONE DAY!

I DIDN'T WANT TO BE overweight I just didn't
consider it a high enough priority to really diet. Oh, a
quick attempt here and there ... but, nothing serious. All
of the diets seemed so expensive or filled with "skinny
food" I knew I wouldn't stay on them, when I had lost 10
pounds, I kept thinking ... "What's the use?"

But, I always looked in the mirror thinking to myself –
"What would I look like if I lost 10-25 pounds? ... what if
my clothes fit a bit better? Oh, that picture really makes
me look heavy from that angle!"

I can assure you ... at a feeling level it was quietly always
on my mind ... I told no one. But, believe me I did not
like being one pound over my IDEAL WEIGHT!

Now, when people ask me, "How did you lose all of
that weight?" and I try to explain the process to them
they typically respond with phrases like, "It can't be that
simple! Oh, I've heard all of this before! I need to lose
weight faster than that!"

I BEG YOU ...
Do not let the simplicity of this diet ... allow you to
dismiss it as "to good to be true".
It is actually working for many people!

Just start using the "THIN THOUGHTS" ... DROP to your "IDEAL WEIGHT" ... and, STAY there.

If you are not ready to start the THINKING MAN Diet ... no one can make you! If you are ready ... no one can stop you ... nothing is standing in your way!

If for some medical reason, you can't lose weight ... I actually have a deep empathy for your situation ... I know somewhat how it feels to have others think you highly undisciplined, when in fact you can do nothing about your weight.

If you aren't ready, at this phase of your life I completely understand ... start the THINKING MAN Diet when you are ready. Sometimes you just can't take on "one more thing!" I've been where you are many times!

If now is the right time for you ... get ready to actually "feel thin" as you approach your "IDEAL WEIGHT"!

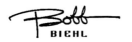
BIEHL

At Your

"IDEAL WEIGHT"

You will not hear

(Or, need to think of yourself as ...)

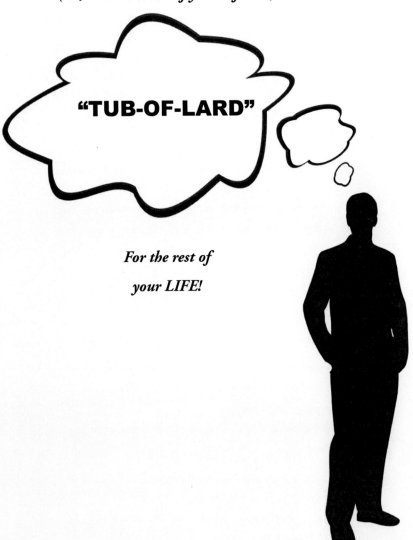

"TUB-OF-LARD"

For the rest of

your LIFE!

CHAPTER 1

UNDERSTANDING
Why "Crash Diets" Work At First, But Don't Last!

MOVING — FROM IMPRESSING OTHERS TO PLEASING YOURSELF!

Many "crash diets" you have seen advertised using thousands of hours of TV commercials, discussed in friendly conversations, read about in magazine articles and even books, and promising "Lose 10 pounds in 10 days" are not focused on you! These advertisers are not focused on helping you "Lose 10 pounds in 10 days". They are focused on helping you impress others! The promise is to help you get ready for the wedding, get ready for the 25th anniversary of your parents, or to attend your high school / college reunion!

"Lose 10 pounds in 10 days" diets are designed to temporarily impress others – not to permanently help you!

It's time you please yourself, not others!

MOVING FROM FOCUSING SHORT TERM TO FOCUSING LONG TERM

The "Lose 10 pounds in 10 days" diet never even attempts to conceal the fact they are focused short term, not long term. There is zero long-term thinking ... just getting you ready for the "big event" coming up shortly! After 10 days of a crash diet, do you honestly think you will keep ordering and using the high-priced "skinny foods" for the rest of your life? When you get sick and tired of the "10-day temporary food" and without new eating habits, do you honestly think your weight will stay off when you go right back to grazing, gobbling, gorging?

It's time you focus on a systematic, logical, lifelong plan and not simply a crash diet!

MOVING FROM "OTHER-ACCOUNTABILITY" TO "SELF-ACCOUNTABILITY"

With many physical fitness and nutritional diets, it is assumed you will join a group of overweight "temporary friends". This approach does help many. They encourage you to allow others to hold you accountable – yet on a temporary basis. So is it any wonder when one leaves that accountability group that their weight comes back?

Once again, this is a huge distinction between the THINKING MAN Diet and pretty much every diet out there! Most diets, "crash diets" especially, are focused on WHO is WATCHING, such as in a group weigh-in. For some people, this "other-accountability" actually helps, but not for the long term. When you are tired of the specific diet food or of having to attend a meeting, the weight comes right back! This is why the THINKING MAN Diet focuses on the fact that NO ONE is watching you – but you! Your friends may not even notice your weight loss at first!

If you are losing weight for YOU, celebrate every single one of those pounds you shed! Do a happy dance when you can tighten your belt another notch, or need a smaller shirt. Let the comments from everyone else just be the icing on your weight loss "cake", instead of the reason for doing it.

The THINKING MAN Diet asks you to commit YOURSELF to changing your thinking. If you have a strong resolve to change your way of thinking, you will be successful! Holding yourself accountable means you will follow the diet even when no one is looking or when it gets rough or when you are really tempted.

If you really do not want to get to your "IDEAL WEIGHT", no one can make you!
If you really want to get to your "IDEAL WEIGHT", no one can stop you!

So ask yourself: Do I want to develop long-term habits of self-accountability?

SATISFIED THINKER

" *I've been around a lot of fitness and nutrition-oriented things over the years, and they ALWAYS focus on external changes to bring about initial change and then hopefully instill a few things that keep people on track. You are focusing entirely on internal changes, which is completely different from anyone else out there. – L.* "

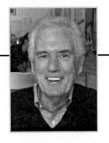

HOW I ACTUALLY FEEL ABOUT: "CRASH DIETS"

I actually FEEL ANGRY about "Lose 10 pounds in 10 days" diets!

Frequently, after a temporary period of time, the man goes right back to eating the same food – in the same amounts as before he started the diet. He continues feeling bad about his self-image, feeling like a failure, feeling he has no self-discipline, and having no long-term hope of staying at the "IDEAL WEIGHT".

The "Lose 10 pounds in 10 days" diets – advertised on every newsstand — never made sense to me. Frankly, they make me ANGRY!

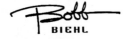

BIEHL

SATISFIED THINKER

"*I think I have read any and every book on the market for diets. I've also paid tons of money for diets. You name it, and I've probably done it. For any diet to be successful, it has to be a lifestyle change, not just a quick fix. This book really hits home. Great job!!!*" – P.

C H A P T E R   2

DECIDING
Your "IDEAL WEIGHT"

REALIZING NO MAN WANTS TO BE ONE POUND OVER HIS "IDEAL WEIGHT"!

Listen to a few heartfelt thoughts from men like yourself:

- "I'd literally give $5,000 today to be able to drop to my "IDEAL WEIGHT" and stay there!"

- "Every time I eat an extra dessert, I feel so guilty – what I wouldn't give for 'guilt free eating'!"

- "When I was young the first word to describe me was 'handsome' … now it's 'overweight / fat'!"

- "Anyone can go on a crash "Lose 10 pounds in 10 days" diet and take it off … but how do I keep it off?"

- "Realistically, I know being overweight is holding me back at work!"

- "I never want to go on a diet again … I just want to learn to eat differently!"

- "I only weigh 15 pounds over what I want to … but that's 15 pounds too much!"

- "I do not want anyone to know I'm on a diet … they will watch every bite I put in my mouth!"

- "I want to eat what everyone else is eating, not be opening a can of 'dandelion greens'!"

Now you no longer have to be one pound overweight!

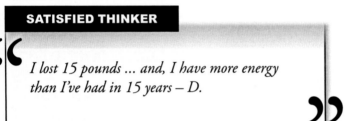

SATISFIED THINKER

I lost 15 pounds ... and, I have more energy than I've had in 15 years – D.

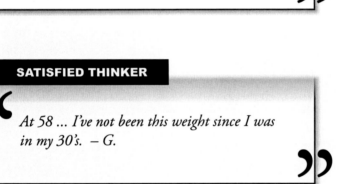

SATISFIED THINKER

At 58 ... I've not been this weight since I was in my 30's. – G.

DECIDING — *Your "IDEAL WEIGHT"*

What is your "IDEAL WEIGHT"? Setting a specific number for my "IDEAL WEIGHT" was actually a huge break through as I started down the path to losing 43 pounds! Today, your "IDEAL WEIGHT" may not be your high school / college playing weight. Considering your age and life situation, Realistically, what is your "IDEAL WEIGHT"?

Most of the men I have chatted with say, "I've actually never thought of defining my "IDEAL WEIGHT" ... I've just wanted to lose ___ pounds!" Most of us have never actually thought of a <u>specific</u> "IDEAL WEIGHT", probably because it seems unattainable. In the past I would frequently think to myself, "You should lose 10-20 pounds!", "You would look better if you lost 5 pounds!", "You would be less embarrassed at the family reunion if you weighted 15 pounds less!" But, I never actually thought about setting an "ideal weight"! 43 pounds was far more than my brain would even entertain. I couldn't imagine losing 43 pounds when I didn't even have the self-discipline to lose 10.

Thin Thought

A key to DROPPING to my IDEAL WEIGHT and STAYING at my IDEAL WEIGHT for LIFE!

I HAVE SET MY "IDEAL WEIGHT" AT _205_ POUNDS!

Sadly, I would always reason like this, "How many pounds should I take off by starving myself, before I can go back to eating 'normally'?"

I remember thinking, "Perhaps I should check with what I 'should weigh' according to some 'scientific' height/weight chart in a doctor's office". I immediately dismissed this idea with the rationalization/realization, "These height/weight charts would show me what someone else should weigh, who has a very different skeletal structure than mine". One of the advantages of the THINKING MAN Diet is that your "IDEAL WEIGHT" is just that ... YOUR "IDEAL".

Setting your "IDEAL WEIGHT" right now will give you something to drive toward, a finish line at the end of your "IDEAL WEIGHT" journey! It is so great to be able to look at your progress, and following these principles will be the first step towards your "IDEAL WEIGHT"! These THIN THOUGHTS will help you form life long habits so you can eat what you love in moderation and still stay at your "IDEAL WEIGHT"!

Go ahead, take a deep breath, and write down your "IDEAL WEIGHT".

Realistically, today my "IDEAL WEIGHT" is _205_ **pounds!**

SATISFIED THINKER

"

The Idea I probably liked best in the entire book was to define my "IDEAL WEIGHT" ... I've lost 15 pounds by thinking different ... you do what you think ... really like the whole idea of "IDEAL WEIGHT"! – D.

"

Setting your "IDEAL WEIGHT" gives you a steady target over a 1 month to 3+ year period (depending on how much weight you have to lose) as you develop consistent "LIFE LONG HABITS" of eating moderately what you enjoy eating to drop to, and stay at your "IDEAL WEIGHT"! To reach your "IDEAL WEIGHT" you may need to lose 250+ pounds ... or, the final 15 you have never been able to lose. Either way THIN THOUGHT number 1 will really help!

SATISFIED THINKER

This is awesome. Today I reached my ideal weight of 180 lbs. (Actually 179.8, down from 180.4 yesterday.)

I set my ideal weight as something I thought was realistic—185, even though my doctor told me years ago I should drop from 190 to 180. But I hadn't been at 180 since I was 35, so I never thought it was possible. It might be helpful for others to set an ideal weight based on where they would be happy.

They can drop it further later.

One other person told me that they had a similar experience. They dropped to an ideal weight, then moved the point lower twice. Honestly, I may go for 175. – S.

Before starting the THINKING MAN Diet, you may want to take a picture of yourself (only for yourself) for motivation so you can accurately see your results. Sometimes it is so hard to see yourself accurately when your body has made such big changes. If you take snapshots of yourself every time you hit a milestone, it will help keep you motivated! Celebrate your progress!

Thin Thought

A key to DROPPING to my IDEAL WEIGHT and STAYING at my IDEAL WEIGHT for LIFE!

2

I HAVE RESET MY "NEVER GO OVER WEIGHT" AT ___ POUNDS

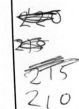

DECIDING — *your "NEVER GO OVER WEIGHT"*

What is your "NEVER GO OVER WEIGHT"? Every man has a weight in his mind he will "NEVER GO OVER"! You have a weight in your mind you will "NEVER GO OVER"! No matter what happens ... no matter how great the temptation you will not allow yourself to go over ___ pounds!

> *My "NEVER GO OVER WEIGHT" is 200 pounds. When I'm 3 pounds under ... I think to myself "I need to back off a bit"!*
>
> *But, when I go over 200 pounds my alarm bell goes off ... it's time to get serious! — S.*

Surprise! It is actually easy to reset your "NEVER GO OVER WEIGHT" to 5-10 pounds over your "IDEAL WEIGHT". Fortunately, once you have reached your "IDEAL WEIGHT" (e.g. 160 pounds) staying between your "IDEAL WEIGHT" and your new "NEVER GO OVER WEIGHT" ... (e.g.160-165) is as easy as staying between your "CURRENT WEIGHT" and your highest "NEVER GO OVER WEIGHT" ... (e.g.195-200).

NEW NORMAL

The term "NEW NORMAL" may be a new term to you. Many men who go on diets keep asking themselves, "When are things going to get back to NORMAL? This is one of the pressing questions of "crash diets". However, what the THINKING MAN Diet is trying to achieve is a LIFESTYLE change where the way we thought about food and eating was the "OLD NORMAL" and the new way of thinking is the "NEW NORMAL" ... actually LIFE LONG / LIFESTYLE HABITS ... our "NEW NORMAL"!

The THINKING MAN Diet is focused on ... long term sustainable habits ... helping you develop a new way of thinking which becomes your "NEW NORMAL"! Thinking of myself as a 160 pound man (not a 195-203 pound man) has become my "NEW NORMAL" ... I don't have to try any more to see myself as a 160 pound man. I never ever think of myself as ever having weighed 203 pounds. This is the depth of change forming a new way of thinking can produce.

And, having 165 pounds as my "NEVER GO OVER WEIGHT" is simply my "NEW NORMAL"!

Depending on your current weight, the THINKING MAN Diet may take a year, or more … focused on establishing new "LIFESTYLE HABITS" of eating the foods you like the very most in moderation … and, establishing a lifestyle that will be both helpful in dropping to your 'IDEAL WEIGHT" and, staying there for the rest of your life!

> The real key is NOT just DROPPING to your "IDEAL WEIGHT" (TAKE IT OFF!)
>
> it is STAYING at your "IDEAL WEIGHT"!
> (KEEP IT OFF!)

Keeping fat off is actually as important (or, more important) than taking fat off. That's why the our slogan is:

> DROPPING to your "IDEAL WEIGHT"
> STAYING at your "IDEAL WEIGHT"!

DO NOT READ ON … until have decided on your NEW "NEVER GO OVER WEIGHT"!

My new "NEVER GO OVER WEIGHT" IS 210 ~~215~~ ~~220~~ pounds.

Guilt free eating! You enjoy no food fully when you are overweight even the tastiest food leaves an aftertaste of guilt. After a certain point food no longer tastes good you are just shoveling it in and the calories just keep adding pounds with no real pleasure!

Your favorite fattening food

> TASTES GREAT ... in your mouth ... for a few seconds!
> TURNS TO GUILT ... in your throat ... for a few seconds!
> TURNS TO FAT ... in your body — for the next 5 days to 5 years!

Experience the "Pure joy of eating" when you are between your "IDEAL WEIGHT" and your "NEVER GO OVER WEIGHT" For the first time you are released to really enjoy eating with no trace of guilt!

Once you actually reach your "IDEAL WEIGHT" and stay between your "IDEAL WEIGHT" and your "NEVER GO OVER WEIGHT" you never have to go on a "DIET" again for the rest of your life! I have found it shockingly easy to stay in this range ... once I got to my "IDEAL WEIGHT" this range has become my "NEW NORMAL"! Today, weighing 160 pounds seems as normal to me as weighing nearly 195 pounds did at my old weight.

SATISFIED THINKER

" *I'm only about 5-10 pounds over my 'IDEAL WEIGHT'". But, when I gain 5 pounds – or, overeat at a family outing – I feel overwhelming guilt for several days. I am using these principles to help me ... get rid of the guilt! – C.* "

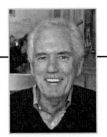

HOW I ACTUALLY FEEL ABOUT:
DECIDING – MY "IDEAL WEIGHT"!

The idea of "IDEAL WEIGHT" really surprised me.

In past years I had always rejected the concept because of some "scientific" IDEAL WEIGHT chart ... which I dismissed immediately because I reasoned, "There skeletal structure is nothing like mine".

But, when it occurred to me I could arbitrarily set my "IDEAL WEIGHT" which would be my very personal diet target for life ... It was a real ... AHA!

Today this idea seems so obvious ... but, it was really a tipping point for me. Defining my "IDEAL WEIGHT" gave me the confidence and focus a fixed target brings! Before my target kept shifting. Before when I'd lose 5 – 10 pounds (comparing my "CURRENT WEIGHT" with my "FORMER WEIGHT" I'd typically celebrate with an 'ice cream cone" ... instead of keeping focused on my "IDEAL WEIGHT".

Frankly, I felt this one thought was a "secret insight" most people never see as a tool for getting to their "IDEAL WEIGHT"!

And, seeing the "NEVER GO OVER WEIGHT" idea was another real AHA! Probably 1,000 times in my life I had reminded myself not to eat another piece of something I really wanted to stay under 200 pounds ... my former "NEVER GO OVER WEIGHT". Now by simply changing my "NEVER GO OVER WEIGHT" to 165 pounds (5 pounds over my "IDEAL WEIGHT" of 160) made all of the sense in the world to me ... and, I feel confident for the first time I have found the secret key to the puzzle of ... a life long "KEEP IT OFF!" formula.

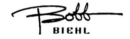
BIEHL

At Your
"IDEAL WEIGHT"

You will not hear
(Or, need to think of yourself as ...)

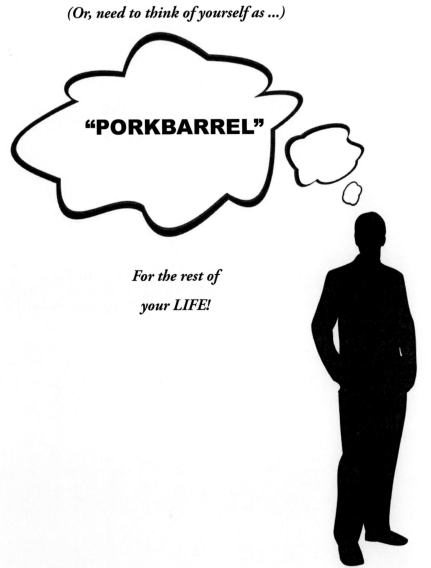

"PORKBARREL"

For the rest of
your LIFE!

CHAPTER 3

THINKING
For Yourself!

Thin Thought

*A key to
DROPPING
to my IDEAL
WEIGHT
and STAYING
at my IDEAL
WEIGHT
for LIFE!*

I

REALLY

WANT TO

GET TO

MY "IDEAL

WEIGHT"

BECAUSE

I can enjoy
this next season of
30 years to
serve others in my domain.

ASKING — *Why Do I Want To Get To My "IDEAL WEIGHT"?*

Think about it: Why do you actually want to weigh less?

✗ K ✗ K

> Without an adequate answer to the question, "Why?", the price of change is always too high!

Unless you have a solid answer to this question ("Why do you want to weigh less?"), you will see the THINKING MAN Diet as just another gimmick and forget about it, just as you may have other diets in the past. Do not do that! Wrestle with this question. Come to grips with it!

So ... <u>WHY?</u>

Even thinking about making change can be scary. You might feel hopeless and despairing because nothing else has worked in the past. Answering the question "WHY?" can take a lot of hard soul searching.

Here are a few thoughts to help you

document your reasoning – right here, right now!

- Today, my "CURRENT WEIGHT" is __240__ pounds.

- I feel like a:

slow, tired, stuffed,
old man, sliding down a hill, no energy

- The reason I really, really, really want to get to my "IDEAL WEIGHT" is …

enjoy my activities w/ energy & feel
great to be with my close friends & be able to
use my gifts w/ others until I die

- If I were at my "IDEAL WEIGHT", I could actually …

Play tennis, have more energy to bring to my
daily tasks, live actively longer, inspire others, look
good, address stress issues w/ food & drink,

- When I get to my "IDEAL WEIGHT", the person I would most like to see me and say, "You have lost weight … you look great!" would be __Dr. Alby__.

- The primary reason I DO NOT want to stay at my current weight is:

cloths don't fit, gluttony & drunkenness not
joints hurt,   pleasing to God!
Poor sex,

In your heart of hearts where no one else sees ... WHY? ...
are you ready to lose weight, at this phase of your life? Like
everything else in life... the THINKING MAN Diet will only
work if you follow it. The only one who will know if you do ... is
you!

Why do you want to weigh less? To be
healthy? To look better naked? To be able
to run and play tag with your kids? So you
are not the "big one"? You don't need to
tell me – or anyone else! But you do need
to be honest with yourself! That honesty
will help you stick to your commitment
regardless of what diets your friends go
on and off of in the meantime! Make
a serious commitment to yourself, and
decide here and now a change must be
made!

"

*For me, keeping it off ... is actually harder ...
but more important than taking it off!"* — S.

"

Thin Thought

*A key to
DROPPING
to my IDEAL
WEIGHT
and STAYING
at my IDEAL
WEIGHT
for LIFE!*

5

**I KNOW
MY
THINKING
IS KEEP-
ING ME
"OVER-
WEIGHT"**

OVERWEIGHT people think "normal" is:

- Always taking seconds
- Getting the biggest piece of pie ... the biggest scoop of ice cream
- Watching games is where everyone is 'pigging out' ... including me!"

"IDEAL WEIGHT" people think "normal" is:

- Never taking seconds
- Getting the smallest piece of pie ... and savoring it!
- Watching games ... one dish of _____ is really as satisfying as X5 dishes!

Consider this reality:

You will see a LOT of really obese people ... often retired early for health reasons in their 60's!

You will see a FEW really obese people ... typically on painful knees / hips in their 70's!

You will see FAR FEWER really obese people … seeing the doctor every other day in their 80's!

You will RARELY see really obese people … in their 90's!

How long do you actually want to live? How long do you actually want to be active with your children, grandchildren, and great grandchildren? You do not want to feel like a huge 18-wheeler semi-truck fully loaded with heavy cargo powered by a tiny car with 4-cylinder engine.

As you walk into a restaurant ... walking by tables ...

- Watch how much the OVERWEIGHT people <u>order</u> ... plates running over!
- Watch how much OVERWEIGHT people <u>actually eat</u> ... clean plates ... wipe, scrape, lick to last drop!

AND ...

- Watch how much the "IDEAL WEIGHT" people <u>actually eat</u> ... sharing, moderation, doggy bags.

You can still eat exactly the foods you want to eat ... you just make your "NEW NORMAL" eating less of it!

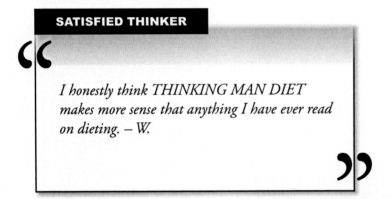

SATISFIED THINKER

I honestly think THINKING MAN DIET makes more sense that anything I have ever read on dieting. – W.

THINKING MORE ABOUT "HOW MUCH" YOU EAT ... THAN "WHAT" YOU EAT!

The THINKING MAN Diet does not tell you WHAT to eat ... it teaches you rather how to SAVOR what you do eat!

The basic premise of the THINKING MAN Diet is you can eat what you choose, and get to your "IDEAL WEIGHT", as long as you follow the THIN THOUGHTS. However, your weight loss will be jumpstarted if you are also monitoring what you choose to put in your body. Eating more vegetables and fruits would be beneficial. Eating less pastries, fried foods, and sugar will help you reach your goal even faster!

You can still eat exactly the foods you want to eat. You just need to make your "NEW NORMAL" eating less of it! The basic change is how much you are eating, not what you eat. Once you make this decision, and with discipline, you can reach your "IDEAL WEIGHT"!

The THINKING MAN Diet does not suggest skipping meals ... just eating less at each meal.

CHANGING – *your thinking from dieting to thin thoughts helps you stay at your IDEAL WEIGHT for life!*

Perhaps I should have called the THINKING MAN Diet the "IDEAL WEIGHT" DIET. But one of the main reasons the THINKING MAN Diet is so successful is the lifelong focus on THIN THOUGHTS.

Think of the THINKING MAN Diet as a LIFESTYLE change. It should not plan to get to your "IDEAL WEIGHT" and then go right back to your old habits. In the THINKING MAN Diet, you are
   • NOT changing WHAT you eat... SHORT TERM

- You are changing HOW YOU THINK about eating and HOW MUCH you eat… LONG TERM.

It's only fair to remind you the THINKING MAN Diet works, but it is not a quick fix! It might take a longer period of time than you would like to get to your "IDEAL WEIGHT". For me it took several months! I know this may not be what you may want to hear. There are going to be days where you'll feel like quitting, or gorging. THAT IS OKAY. There are going to be difficult days – everyone has them. The THINKING MAN Diet can still work for you, even when things are hard in other areas of your life. But the next day … get back on your trusted scales!

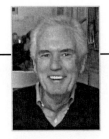

HOW I ACTUALLY FEEL ABOUT:
"THINKING … FOR MYSELF! "

My personal "tipping point" was the very sad thought that I may not be around to enjoy my children, grandchildren, and great grandchildren in their later years if I continued being overweight!

- You will see a LOT of really obese people … often retired early for health reasons in their 60's!
- You will see a FEW really obese people … typically on troubled knees / hips in their 70's!
- You will see FAR FEWER really obese people … seeing the doctor every other day in their 80's!
- You will RARELY see really obese people … in their 90's!

I have never liked the feeling of having others tell me what I can and cannot eat ... even for a few months at a time. To tell me what I can eat and what I can't eat or how much I need to exercise ... NO WAY! But to show me how to eat differently to get to my "IDEAL WEIGHT" ... great!

I'm willing to eat LESS real butter, pancakes, Canadian maple syrup, popcorn when I see it is far better for me to eat less of these favorites for my long-term health ... just don't tell me I can't eat them any more (unless of course it is proven to be life-threatening).

Bob
BIEHL

At Your

"IDEAL WEIGHT"

You will not hear

(Or, need to think of yourself as ...)

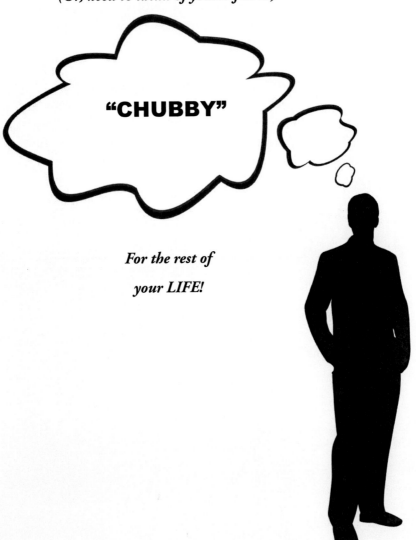

For the rest of

your LIFE!

CHAPTER 4

WEIGHING
Yourself Every Morning!

WEIGHING *Yourself — Every morning ... naked!*

Thin Thought

A key to DROPPING to my IDEAL WEIGHT and STAYING at my IDEAL WEIGHT for LIFE!

I WEIGH MYSELF NAKED EVERY MORNING!

Another important key to the THINKING MAN Diet is weighing in EVERY MORNING. I know this might go against other dietary advice you have heard, and many people suggest weighing yourself once a week is sufficient. I disagree! If you wait that long, it's possible you have a GREAT day, and then you don't try as hard all week. It's also possible you have a HORRIBLE day, and you get depressed for the rest of the week and want to eat more ice cream! There is no accountability on those other days of the week, and your weight stays the same or goes up!

If you weigh yourself EVERY day, whether the scale "looks happy or sad", you know exactly where you are in relationship to your "IDEAL WEIGHT"!

When I weigh myself on a daily basis, it is far easier to have the discipline to trim a bit here and there, and to go back down a pound or two. NO ONE wants to RE-

LOSE weight! You worked so hard to take it off – don't let it go back up because you didn't weigh in daily!

NAKED. I know when you have weight to lose, "NAKED" can feel like a dirty word. It may be the last thing you want to do. But it is so important to weigh yourself naked to get your accurate weight. PLUS, there is nothing to add more weight! It may feel uncomfortable at first, but take a look at your body before you step on the scale. It is so great to see it change! If you stay the course and follow your THIN THOUGHTS, you will begin to see real change in the way you look. After you reach your "IDEAL WEIGHT", you will reach a point where you are happy with what you see in the mirror, even if it isn't "perfect" according to some imaginary perfectionistic movie star standard. That is the beauty of the THINKING MAN Diet: Each of us has our own IDEAL.

SATISFIED THINKER

"

Frankly, it has taken me some time getting used to seeing the "new face" in my mirror ... since I've lost 35 pounds! — E.

"

As you travel, you may find weighing in daily impractical, or impossible. If so, just weigh yourself each morning when you have a scale available.

Thin Thought

A key to DROPPING to my IDEAL WEIGHT and STAYING at my IDEAL WEIGHT for LIFE!

I WEIGH MYSELF ON A "RELIABLE SET OF SCALES"!

WEIGHING ON A SCALE YOU TRUST!

It is important to trust your scales, or you will simply dismiss added weight as the scale's error for the day! This sounds too simple to be important. IT IS NOT! If you don't trust your scales, you will put off weighing for days at a time (a major mistake) and rationalize your weight gain as a problem with your scales more than a problem with your "eating habits". One way to look at the THINKING MAN Diet is you are taking the money you would have been spending on an expensive (nutritional diet) blender and buying scales you trust.

Once you reach your "IDEAL WEIGHT", you can savor a bit more of your favorite food with no trace of guilt or worry. If your scales go up a pound or two some morning, you will simply cut back in some area for a day or two and you get right between your "IDEAL WEIGHT" and your "NEVER-GO-OVER WEIGHT" again!

Everyone slips. But do not quit! Get right back on the scales as soon as possible. You will find eventually the pounds just come off and stay off. THIN THOUGHT 8 helps you stay in the safety range between your "IDEAL WEIGHT" and your "NEVER-GO-OVER WEIGHT"! Start seeing your private mirror and your private scales as your "secret smiling friends", not your "harshest secret critics"!

SATISFIED THINKER

My bathroom scales have become my very private accountability partner ... I don't need a group! – L.

On a vacation, my goal was to not gain more than 2 lbs. There are times when you are going to be eating in restaurants for weeks, and you are going to be having food you love. Setting a goal to not gain more than X lbs. allows you to still use the principles and feel like you succeeded. As soon as you return home, start on your way back down again. – W.

Because the THINKING MAN Diet is a lifestyle, there are going to be times when you really have to be intentional about your THIN THOUGHTS. For instance, if you are vacationing in a beautiful, faraway place, like Switzerland, it would be a CRIME not to have some delightfully delicious Swiss chocolate … and you might never have that opportunity again! Instead of going crazy and eating as much as you want, decide before you go. Allow yourself to indulge, in MODERATION. If you want to try some chocolate – go for it! BUT make sure you are making SMART decisions about how much you are putting into your body. Recognize there are times when you will want to indulge a bit, and if you slip, refocus on the principles as soon as you return. Just because you are on vacation doesn't mean the principles don't apply!

COMPARING YOUR "CURRENT WEIGHT" TO YOUR "IDEAL WEIGHT"

THIN THOUGHT 9 was a huge breakthrough for me in "TAKING OFF AND KEEPING OFF 43 POUNDS"!

Every morning

> compare your
> "CURRENT WEIGHT"
> to your
> "IDEAL WEIGHT"

instead of

> comparing your
> "CURRENT WEIGHT"
> to your
> "FORMER WEIGHT"!

When you compare your "CURRENT WEIGHT" to your "FORMER WEIGHT", you are tempted to "celebrate" and eat a huge scoop of 'rocky road' ice cream!

When you compare your "CURRENT WEIGHT" with your "IDEAL WEIGHT", you are aware of the fact that you are either making progress toward your "IDEAL WEIGHT" (although you still have a ways to go) or you are right on track!

Once you have reached your "IDEAL WEIGHT" and you are under your "NEVER-GO-OVER WEIGHT", you can eat a

---

Thin Thought

A key to DROPPING to my IDEAL WEIGHT and STAYING at my IDEAL WEIGHT for LIFE!

I ALWAYS COMPARE MY "CURRENT WEIGHT" TO MY "IDEAL WEIGHT".

cookie or two with zero guilt, without fear of being in trouble, knowing you will get back on the scales tomorrow, and if you are over your "NEVER-GO-OVER WEIGT", you will trim back the next few days!

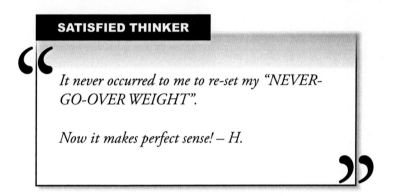

SATISFIED THINKER

It never occurred to me to re-set my "NEVER-GO-OVER WEIGHT".

Now it makes perfect sense! – H.

THIS REALLY WORKS!

quick tip: FROM A HELPFUL READER

When you told me not to compare myself to my starting weight, but to think about how far I have to go to get to my ideal weight, I thought you meant something that you never mention in this book. I felt it was one of the biggest helps to me. In addition to the daily weigh-in, I looked at myself naked in the mirror every morning. I was often amazed at how much thinner I looked. But then I would remind myself to notice how much fat was still there. I would imagine how much better I might look at my ideal weight. I would take about 30 seconds to look from different angles. This was highly motivational to me. It is the one single reason why I said I might push for 175. That's because I can still pinch two inches. And I imagine what 5 more pounds gone might look like. It's why I went to 180 after I achieved my original goal of 185. I thought this was part of your advice, but I guess I just read that into your general principle "don't just think of how much you've lost, think of how much more you need to lose to get to your ideal weight. — S.

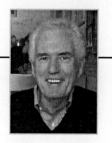

HOW I ACTUALLY FEEL ABOUT:
WEIGHING — EVERY MORNING

Comparing my "CURRENT WEIGHT" to my "IDEAL WEIGHT" seems like a simple thought. But this is a discipline, which keeps me day after day focused on STAYING at my "IDEAL WEIGHT".

This may be one of the top 3 thoughts in the THINKING MAN Diet!

It felt great to look forward to "my very private weigh-in" each morning and see my weight dropping in a regular pattern toward my "IDEAL WEIGHT"! It feels great now to get on the scales at my "my very private weigh in" each morning and see my weight consistently staying between my "IDEAL WEIGHT" and my "NEVER-GO-OVER WEIGHT"!

Before, when I didn't have a trustworthy scale, in all honesty, I'd rationalize, telling myself, "It was the scales. I hadn't really gained 2 pounds yesterday because of all the food I had gobbled." It feels great now to know exactly where I am. I'm not trying to fool myself. Here is where I actually am!

When I slip (I'm embarrassed to admit it but I do!), I have come to feel pleasure in getting back on the scales ASAP! I committed to never go over my "NEVER-GO-OVER WEIGHT" again. So when I do slip, weighing myself each and every morning until I'm back to my "IDEAL WEIGHT" gives me great comfort, knowing I have a proven process for getting right back to my "IDEAL WEIGHT"!

Another "tipping point" insight: Getting back on the scales is frankly where my stopping (in the past) most frequently occurred. If I knew I had gained weight again, I'd put off climbing the "huge hill" of getting back on the scales – it seemed 100 feet high, not 1.5 inches. When I committed (in my heart where no one else sees) to getting back on the scales every day for "my very private weigh-in" (always comparing with my "ideal weight") for the rest of my life, regardless of how I felt about it, it has become a real confidence builder ... AHA!

Bobb

BIEHL

CHAPTER 5

SAVORING
Every Bite!

LEARNING TO SAVOR YOUR FIRST BITE!

Often we take words like SAVOR for granted at a very shallow level. Here are a few examples of the usage of the word SAVOR which helps highlight the delight you should take in the very first bite of anything you are eating:

- He savored the aroma of the baking pies.

- They savored every last morsel of food.

- She was just savoring the moment.

- The team is still savoring its victory.

- He savored the memories of his vacation.

Get in the habit of SAVORING YOUR FIRST BITE of anything you eat. It will help you stay at your "IDEAL WEIGHT"! The first bite always tastes the very best, and every bite beyond the first one tastes less and less great!

Thin Thought

A key to DROPPING to my IDEAL WEIGHT and STAYING at my IDEAL WEIGHT for LIFE!

10

I SAVOR MY FIRST BITE!

This is what I refer to as "BOBB'S LAW OF DIMINISHING PLEASURE"!

Try a personal experiment on your very next meal. Savor each and every bite. The first bite is the best! Bite by bite, think about each bite ... how good it tastes, how it feels in your mouth, listening to friends talking while you are savoring bite after bite. After a few savored bites, you will begin experiencing "BOBB'S LAW OF DIMINISHING PLEASURE" even with your very favorite foods.

SATISFIED THINKER

"

You are exactly right. It doesn't take many bites of even my favorite foods to actually begin experiencing the "Law of Diminishing Pleasure"! – R.

"

"
I cannot believe the savoring pleasure I'm getting out of my first bite of anything ... just by stopping to think about it! – P.
"

Taste is what your mouth is craving, not volume. Better one bite of what you really want than a plateful of what you don't! A simple taste of your very favorite ice cream is what your mouth is craving, not 15 scoops of it. Learn to stay on the one spoonful end of the journey, not on the 15 scoops. Your first taste is actually what your body is really after!

Imagine with me for just one minute YOUR VERY FAVORITE FOOD:

First bite = TASTES FANTASTIC!

Next 10 =   still tastes very satisfying ...
Next 10 =   you're still thinking, "This is really good ... but I'm beginning to feel satisfied ..."
Next 50 =   getting tired of this ...
Next 50 =   stuffed ... had enough ...
Next 50 =   never want to see it again!

This is an extreme but accurate example of "BOBB'S LAW OF DIMINISHING PLEASURE"!

" *I have never really been on diet so I may not have the ideal perspective, but the discipline aspect I really connect with. Since I am allergic to wheat, I am a lot more aware of what food does to me. It forces me to select specific foods, portions ... It also allows me to savor things differently. (For example, since most pizza dough is made from wheat, I can't eat it. Recently many pizza places have started serving gluten-free pizza. For the first time in a long while, I can eat pizza again. I sure enjoy it now.) I think the routine of eating takes away the value of what is being eaten sometimes. – L.* "

Thin Thought

*A key to
DROPPING
to my IDEAL
WEIGHT
and STAYING
at my IDEAL
WEIGHT
for LIFE!*

I MAKE

SURE MY

FOOD

TASTES

GREAT ...

OR I

DO NOT

EAT IT!

No one wants to be stuck eating cardboard-tasting food, and if you do eat it just to lose weight, it probably won't become your 30-year LIFESTYLE! Make sure your food TASTES GREAT or DO NOT EAT IT! Why put something in your body you don't enjoy? Make sure every single one of those bites is worth the calories!

If you enjoy French fries, like I do, make this a personal game with yourself: Think carefully and rate every piece to see the actual number of delicious fries you can really enjoy. It may be far fewer than you think! Remember to use your THIN THOUGHT principles. Play a game with yourself, and SAVOR your fries.

Sometimes they are cold ...
   DO NOT EAT THEM ... leave them!

Sometimes they are overdone ...
   DO NOT EAT THEM ... leave them!

Sometimes they are too greasy ...
   DO NOT EAT THEM ... leave them!

See how many calorie-packed fries you can leave on your plate! Your friends will never even notice how many fries you leave on your plate or in your basket. Enjoy the taste of your fries. Don't make gorging on them one of your "lifelong habits" – or your belt size!

There is a famous television personality who always orders

"exactly 5 fries" with his burger. That way, he savors each bite of every one of those 5 fries! If that would help you, go for it! If not, play the mental game "LEAVE SOME"! If they are delicious, enjoy as many as you like and leave as many as you can at the end of your meal!

Your new THINKING MAN lifestyle is about SAVORING taste, not GOBBLING volume!

Thin Thought

A key to
DROPPING
to my IDEAL
WEIGHT
and STAYING
at my IDEAL
WEIGHT
for LIFE!

I

DO NOT

GRAZE
(eat endlessly)

GOBBLE
(eat without

thinking)

GORGE
(eat after satisfied)

EATING SLOWLY GIVES YOU A CHANCE TO ASK YOURSELF:

O   AM I "GRAZING"?
           (Grazing ... feeds fat!)

O   AM I "GOBBLING"?
           (Gobbling ... feeds fat!)

O   AM I "GORGING"
           (Gorging ... feeds fat!)

Where does your body store fat: double chin ... waist ... legs?

When you eat until you are satisfied, you are feeding yourself.

When you start GRAZING, GOBBLING, GORGING, you are feeding your fat!

Reducing your eating speed gives you time to think. Monitor yourself very carefully:

- Am I really enjoying this food? If not, I won't eat it!
- Am I getting full? If so, I'll stop eating it –
  and I'll ask for a "doggy bag"!

If you eat more slowly, you'll eat far less. If you eat slowly, you won't keep eating when others finish. Over a lifetime, you will actually eat far less, making it far easier to stay at your "IDEAL WEIGHT"!

SATISFIED THINKER

As my wife and I were savoring our dinner together, we discovered another benefit of eating more slowly – communication! Rather than just sitting down and eating so we can get on with the day, as we savored each bite, we had more time to talk.

Also, she is going to make a little table tent to put on the table: Savor Each Bite. – R.

As an additional bonus: When you do not GRAZE, GOBLE, GORGE, you will have far less heartburn! ☺

Three lifetime bad habits every man, woman, and child should break once and for all: GRAZING, GOBBLING, and GORGING!

"GRAZING" is ...
   having an "unlimited supply" of anything fattening
   constantly available ... and nibbling at it!

Examples:

1. An open bag or jar of any form of candy ... available!
2. An open box of crackers, chips, and snacks ... available!
3. A whole pie, cake, other desserts on the counter with a spoon / fork in it ... available!

You just walk past and take another piece, take another sip, etc. GRAZING is something we all do ... and we can all STOP! If you never START it again, you will never DO it again!

Stay far away from an "unlimited supply" of anything like candy, desserts, snacks, tempting you to keep nibbling / GRAZING all day. Cows graze all day. Enough said?

What is your very favorite food? Let's say chocolate ... or nuts ... or candy. You can add many pounds a year just by grazing on these favorites. So, when you decide to have a "few nuts", put a few in a dish and when they are gone, you are done! Eat no snack from the container. It is an endless supply. Before you know it, the entire container is gone. The same with a pint / quart of ice cream or a large bag of potato chips or a new package of cookies or a fresh-out-of-the-oven anything! NO GRAZING!

One of the great things about the THINKING MAN Diet is that you can eat at parties! You don't have to look for the low fat or stick to just vegetables or avoid the dip. What is important is you take a moderately sized portion, such as a few chips, and when you are done, you are DONE! So if you only get that few chips, really SAVOR them! There is no need to feel different, or awkward; you only need to be mentally prepared! Do NOT stand by the bowl full of food – it will only tempt you to help yourself to more!

At home, it is also really helpful to look at serving sizes. If you portion out a smaller amount, it will stop you from eating the entire gallon of ice cream or the whole bag of chips! This new shift in your thinking about eating will help you get to your "IDEAL WEIGHT" and stop you from putting on pounds over time.

It is important to mention the counterpart to our food choices: drinks. It may seem strange to think of GRAZING in terms of drinks, but really, we GRAZE with drinks all the time! Because we sip on things all day long, it is easy to forget the effect they have on our weight. With the THINKING MAN Diet, I am not suggesting you restrict what you drink – only that you be mindful of them. If you are the type of person who drinks many sodas in a day, it could be affecting your weight loss. If you want to have a drink, great! However, moderate the amount of drinks you have and make sure you are thinking about what you put into your body.

It also begs to be said that if you are trying to improve your health, it is better to have a healthy snack, such as fruit, over chocolate. But that is entirely up to you! If you are going to graze, consider grazing on (have constantly available) healthy fruits, not fattening sweets!

> *I really noticed the "THINKING MAN" advantage the last time I ate at my favorite Mexican restaurant. Before, without thinking I'd have "grazed" down 1-2 baskets of chips and salsa (hundreds of calories). I ate a few chips with my friends, and not one friend noticed I'd changed my "grazing" habits. – 0.*

GOBBLING is ...
eating (usually eating fast) without thinking about what you are eating!

Examples of GOBBLING are EATING WHILE ...

Watching TV,
Reading the newspaper,
Hurrying to catch a plane, train, bus ...
Anything that allows you to keep shoveling down the calories
While not really ever enjoying them!

There should be a sign beside each bowl, plate, or dish, "THOU SHALT NOT GOBBLE!"

If I am in a hurry to finish and to get back to work or to catch a plane or to meet a friend, I tend to gobble! Rushed food adds just as many calories to our bodies – and very little pleasure.

Go ahead and eat snacks – but not while concentrating on your favorite TV program or thinking about ball games or anything else! It is not wise to be stuffing calories while watching TV and thinking about the program, not what's going into your mouth and becoming part of your ever-widening body.

When you do eat foods like potato chips, don't down them by the fistful. Consider breaking up the chips. Just ¼ of a chip will give you the taste of a whole chip with your sandwich, but not the calories of an entire chip. Leave chips on your plate ... no one will even notice!

The THINKING MAN Diet is a change in your thinking. Tell yourself: "If I am in a hurry to finish and I AM GOBBLING, then I need to leave it!" Remember rushed food and drinks add just as many calories to your body, and, very, very, little pleasure! Take pleasure in eating slowly, and you will also be able to take pleasure in seeing the scale go down!

Never start grazing or gobbling, so you will never have to stop it again!

quick tip: FROM A HELPFUL READER

Always putting our fork down between bites helps us gobblers! – PS

GORGING is ...
   eating even after you are <u>satisfied</u>!

Have you ever eaten so much your stomach ached, but then still took another bite? I'm embarrassed to admit I have many times! I'd feel stuffed but because the others around me ordered dessert, I did too! That is GORGING! Just because others are still eating does not mean you need join them! Stop and think. LISTEN to your body and don't GORGE just to be polite! If you really wanted dessert, eat one savoring bite! Don't continue to eat (or drink) after you are full.

SATISFYING YOURSELF — <u>NEVER</u> FEELING "FULL" AND "STUFFED"!

It is crucial to the THINKING MAN Diet mindset that you NEVER EAT JUST BECAUSE IT'S IN FRONT OF YOU! It sounds way too simple to be helpful, but often we eat just because it's in front of us, or because we have made it a "bad habit", i.e. because others are eating or just to be polite or just because we always have it at this time of day. Don't fall into this trap! For instance, when you sit down at night, really think about how you are feeling. If you are hungry, by all means have a small snack! But if you are SATIFIED, <u>DON'T EAT ANY MORE!</u>

Thin Thought

*A key to
DROPPING
to my IDEAL
WEIGHT
and STAYING
at my IDEAL
WEIGHT
for LIFE!*

13

**I HATE
FEELING
FULL OR
STUFFED...
WHEN I'M
SATIFIED,
I STOP!**

Most of us don't really think about avoiding the feeling of being stuffed before it happens. Usually what we are eating is so tasty we keep wanting more! Before we know it, we have eaten way more than we need and then we feel STUFFED. BUT with the THINKING MAN Diet, as long as we are simply AWARE of the possibility, we can change our thinking about eating. Being STUFFED never needs be a reality again.

The best mental picture I can give you of stuffed is what most Americans do at Thanksgiving. We are so excited for the turkey and the cranberry sauce and the stuffing, so we load our plate! We dig in and we eat quickly – pardon the pun, but we technically "gobble" on the turkey! Then we realize we forgot the mashed potatoes and corn, so we pile it on! By the time we are finished eating, we want to lie down or unbutton our pants because we are so uncomfortable – and there is still pie! Who can turn down pumpkin pie that's covered completely over with real whipped cream? By the time we are done, our stomach is in pain and we vow not to do it again ... until next year!

Does this mental picture help you to put an image to the term STUFFED? Who wants to feel that way? Not me! But if we had used our THIN THOUGHTS, and evaluated how hungry we were, taken a smaller portion, really SAVORED each bite, eaten slowly so you didn't GOBBLE, didn't graze on snacks beforehand, and stopped when we were full, it could have been a much better meal! We would be closer to our "IDEAL WEIGHT" and feeling great, while everyone else is on the couch groaning!

Now that you can visualize STUFFED, you can AVOID it! Let's learn to enjoy the PLEASURE of NOT feeling stuffed, even more than the DISPLEASURE of feeling stuffed for hours after gorging!

A key to understanding the term STUFFED is to define it. In the THINKING MAN Diet, we use a continuum to put "STUFFED" into perspective.

Bobb's SATISFACTION CONTINUUM

Actually starving! (Bulimic)	Feels like ... "I'm Starving!"	Hungry	It's time to eat ... so let's eat.	Satisfied	Full	Stuffed	Miserable Stuffed!

The slower you eat, the higher the likelihood of you asking yourself,

"Am I actually satisfied? If so, it's time to stop!

or

"Am I past satisfied and on to FULL, STUFFED, MISERABLY STUFFED?"
If so, then I'm grazing, gobbling, gorging ... and becoming fatter and fatter!

For most men, the idea there could be so many spaces on the satisfied continuum is shocking! We tend to think, "I am hungry" or "I am full". In reality there are many more than just those two! Sadly there are people who experience true hunger because there is actually nothing to eat. Eating very little for a couple days does not capture the severity of TRUE hunger. Most of us have never been truly HUNGRY in our lives!

To benefit from the THINKING MAN Diet, you should ideally be between the four middle spaces on the continuum at all times. You don't want to get to the point where you feel you are STARVING, because it will set you up for GOBBLING or GORGING! You also don't want to get past the point of comfortably FULL to avoid getting to STUFFED!

By eating slowly and SAVORING, you are able to stay in the middle of the continuum. You will have a chance to evaluate whether you are actually SATISFIED … and if so, STOP! Every single bite beyond SATISFIED is actually GORGING. GORGING is one of the main reasons so many men struggle with reaching their "IDEAL WEIGHT"!

SATISFIED THINKER

> *The THINKING MAN DIET moved me from "JUST EATING" to thinking about the critical difference between feeling "SATISFIED" and feeling "FULL".*
>
> *I now hate the feeling of being "full" or "stuffed"! – S.*

An old English nursery rhyme:

> It's a very odd thing,
> as odd as can be,
> That whatever she eats,
> turns into Miss T.

When you are satisfied ... STOP!

Try going to bed feeling a bit hungry. You have likely heard the great advice:

> Eat a big breakfast (eat like a KING) ...
>> Eat a healthy lunch (eat like a QUEEN) ...
>>> Eat an early ½ dinner (eat like a PAUPER)
>>>> Eat nothing (very little) after 8:00 p.m. ... ideally!

Understand these are rules of thumb. This is not a set of rigid rules! Some days you may have a small breakfast and attend a huge dinner in the evening! But over the next 30 years, the above is your healthiest pattern. Make "a big breakfast, a healthy lunch, an early dinner, very little after 8:00" a LIFESTYLE HABIT!

Our bodies burn calories and fat even while we are asleep! Instead of making your body work extra hard to burn the food you ate just before you went to bed, why not let it burn your fat! This will help you reach your "IDEAL WEIGHT"!

Here is a challenge: Try going to bed just a bit hungry for 5 days. I bet you will never want to go to bed full or stuffed again! It will actually feel good to tuck yourself into bed feeling somewhat hungry, knowing the scale will be closer to (or at) your "IDEAL WEIGHT" in the morning!

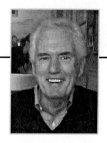

HOW I ACTUALLY FEEL ABOUT:
SAVORING ... EVERY BITE!

Very few people actually SAVOR even the most exotic foods ... which is a TRAGEDY!

I love the taste of pancakes with real butter and real Canadian maple syrup. I have this combination several times a month. I may only have ½ a pancake per breakfast but I have it "just the way I like it!"

Learning to SAVOR each bite was a real tipping point for me, especially SAVORING the first bite. Yes, I do experience "Bobb's Law of Diminishing Pleasure" even when I eat my very favorite pancakes.

I have learned to SAVOR my first bite of pancakes before anything else, then SAVOR one bite of ham/sausage, then

SAVOR one bite of egg, then I SAVOR the taste of all three together – knowing I will eat like a king at breakfast so I won't need as much later in the day.

Learning to eat slowly (coming from a family of "lightning-fast eaters") has been difficult for me. But it is what allows me to experience the REAL pleasure of eating – not just grazing, gobbling, or gorging! In the past – and honestly occasionally still – I have been very guilty of grazing, gobbling and gorging! But eating slower has given me the ability to actually SAVOR my food and with "new eyes" watch others continue grazing, gobbling and gorging ... with apparently zero SAVORING of the calories they are gobbling!

Experiencing the "tipping point" between being satisfied and being full has made a world of difference on how I feel about eating less as I move toward (and now stay) at my "IDEAL WEIGHT"!

I have developed a few new pleasures in life: going to bed a bit hungry, leaving food on my plate, cutting fries into ¼ their size and leaving as many as possible, savoring, feeling thin, fitting in my clothing ... rather than the temporary pleasure of grazing, gobbling, or gorging!

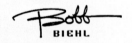

BIEHL

CHAPTER 6

EATING AND DRINKING
Whatever You Want, Just Less Of It!

Thin Thought

*A key to
DROPPING
to my IDEAL
WEIGHT
and STAYING
at my IDEAL
WEIGHT
for LIFE!*

I TAKE A

MODER-

ATE SIZE

HELPING ...

FIRST

SERVING!

TAKING A MODERATE SIZE HELPING THE FIRST TIME!

Make a lifelong habit of taking a MODERATE-SIZE portion of whatever you really enjoy eating – the FIRST TIME it's passed! No one is watching how large or small a helping you take the first time the delicious potatoes come around at breakfast, lunch, or dinner. No one is watching how large or small a helping you take of potato salad at a favorite buffet, church potluck, or family picnic. They only watch if your plate is dripping off the sides! From now on, form a new LIFELONG HABIT of taking a moderate-size portion of whatever you really want and SAVORING EACH BITE!

Consider the power of a new "moderation lifestyle" lifelong habit.

Get in a few new habits, e.g. always ordering:

> 1 egg, not 2
> 2 strips of bacon, not 4
> 1 pancake, not 2-4 ... this is plenty to satisfy!

Is it obvious to you what difference just this one single habit will make in the next 10 years?

No need to be obsessed with calorie counting. Just form the new habit of ordering and eating less!

Perhaps, order one pancake and immediately cut it in half because you enjoy the taste of pancakes but not eat all the calories of a whole order of pancakes. You can still add lots of real butter and real syrup but only on half of a pancake, not 2-4. Eating half of a pancake gives your mouth the same taste as a mouth packed full, but without a stomach crammed with the calories 2-4 pancakes contain. Even if the meal comes with 3 pancakes, tell them you want just one.

At home, it is also important to pay attention to portion sizes. In a restaurant or at a friend's house, you are at the mercy of what you are served; at home, you are in control. In the past, when I wanted a snack, I would get myself a bowl of ice cream. I didn't consider myself a GORGER; after all, I didn't eat two or three bowls! I simply got my bowl and filled it. But the problem is there are many different sizes of bowls! I was actually eating 2 or 3 times the serving size, while patting myself on the back for my restraint! Although my new "much smaller" bowl seemed pitifully small at first, it really helped me to portion out exactly what the serving size called for. I'm not going to lie – I lick the ice cream scoop clean ... but I only have a small dish and really SAVORED it. I still have my ice cream, and I am still able to stay at my "IDEAL WEIGHT".

Thin Thought

*A key to
DROPPING
to my IDEAL
WEIGHT
and STAYING
at my IDEAL
WEIGHT
for LIFE!*

I NEVER

TAKE

"SECONDS"!

RESISTING THE TEMPTATION OF TAKING "SECONDS" ON ANYTHING!

Approximately <u>50%</u> of the pleasure of eating is in the <u>FIRST BITE</u>!

Approximately <u>90%</u> of the pleasure is in the <u>FIRST SERVING!</u>

The second serving contains "lots" of extra calories, but a vastly diminished pleasure. It feels more like shoveling it in, gorging, stuffing. Simply smile and say, "No, thank you, it was delicious but I'm feeling very satisfied at the moment!" Don't let anyone pressure you into taking "seconds"!

I know it might seem like simple common sense, but not taking second helpings is a huge thinking shift in the THINKING MAN Diet. This one simple lifelong HEALTHY HABIT will play a major role in helping you stay at your "IDEAL WEIGHT"! This is a simple one-time commitment to make a lifelong habit of NEVER TAKING SECONDS! Once made, this key will help you reach your "IDEAL WEIGHT" and no friends will ever notice. I used to take seconds constantly. If I still felt at all hungry (which, if I am honest, wasn't really hunger) or if the food was good, I simply wanted more! Instead, I should have been focused on really ENJOYING what I had on my plate, and going to bed less than full. When you COMMIT to NO SECONDS as a lifestyle, it will really make a huge difference!

Most of the time, the second serving doesn't even taste that great by the end, so why do we feel the need to eat it? If the food is that great, then make it again … or you can always order it again in a restaurant or have it another time. There is no reason to GORGE!

Serving up plates before bringing them to the table, instead of placing the food in the center of the table, is a practical way to avoid a second helping. It is much easier to avoid having more if the food is not right in front of you. If you have to work for it, you are much more likely to stick to just one helping.

EATING YOUR FAVORITE DESSERTS –
ASKING FOR A "SMALLER" SERVING BEFORE IT IS SERVED!

The THINKING MAN Diet is not about denying yourself. If someone tells us we CAN'T have something, we just crave it MORE! This diet doesn't tell you to eliminate desserts, because it's a lifestyle change! The THINKING MAN Diet will help you reach your goal and maintain it, while still eating dessert! The key is moderation.

If you are at a friend's home for dinner, tell the host / hostess you would prefer a small piece of dessert BEFORE it is served. (Be careful of this one if it's your MAMA!) That way, he/she won't be insulted if you don't gorge on a huge piece. Say, "I don't sleep well if I have too much sugar late at night." He/she will understand and will not feel insulted!

Be very careful not to insult the person who is the cook/baker. If you do not know the host/hostess well, you may not want to use this approach. Use your wise judgment as to when to use this principle and when to just go ahead and eat whatever is served.

Take the smaller piece, SAVOR THE DESSERT, savor smaller bites, and do not gobble! Pace yourself to end when those with large pieces end as they gobble with huge, high-calorie, way-overweight bites. In reality your first three bites will actually cure your dessert craving! The rest is pure calories! Sugar turns to fat and disturbs your sleep at the same time – double trouble!

My sister, Jann Bach, imagines her 2-3 bites of any dessert to be the last 2-3 bites available. She finds it is much more satisfying. Try it!

This would be a good place to chat about the need to stop seeing "super sugar" food as the "ultimate reward / celebration"! In many families, the primary reward for a "job well done" is an ice cream cone, a hot fudge sundae, a cookie, a piece of pie and ice cream. Food has become the ultimate way to celebrate some major achievement. Reward yourself with something other than food ... or reward yourself by savoring a very small dish of ice cream, much smaller than you would normally eat!

At the end of a "Lose 10 pounds in 10 days" crash diet, what is the most typical activity? You guessed it! Let's go celebrate with a big helping of what we have been "starving for" for the last 10 days, now that the "event" is over!

Learn to celebrate with something other than MORE FOOD! Instead, reward yourself with some new clothes you can now fit into, a trip, a boat ride, or maybe even a deeply savored cup of tea / coffee – something other than a huge dish of ice cream with hot fudge, whipped cream, and a cherry on the top!

Stop rewarding yourself primarily with food (especially desserts)!

" *You are focusing entirely on internal changes, which is completely different from most others out there.*

Your other 10+ books about Leadership and Management deals with internal change for improvement. Because of this fact, this book feels like it fits right in to what you have been doing all along.

I liked how you blended the idea of weight management with the mind. You didn't lay out a calorie intake plan or protein versus carbs versus sugar versus something else. Totally different approach. – J. "

quick tip: FROM A HELPFUL READER

Actually, it was a lighthearted competition that was finally the thing that got me started. Other things may be a way to get you started but you will only succeed long term if you have a good answer to the question "Why?" – P.

Loopholes are dangerous. A few years ago, I think I would have been crowned "King of Diet Loopholes"!

If you are trying to order one pancake and the order comes with three, it is NOT an excuse to eat more. YOU must be personally committed to your "IDEAL WEIGHT" if you want it to work. Instead of saying, "Oh, well," and continuing your bad habits, YOU change them!

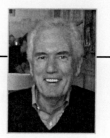

HOW I ACTUALLY FEEL ABOUT:
EATING AND DRINKING --
WHATEVER I WANT, JUST
LESS OF IT!

Focus for a minute on two words:
    OFFEND and DISCIPLINED.

When eating, I really don't want to feel like I'm offending anyone at any time!

At the same time, I do want to be disciplined in my eating habits.

Taking a moderate-size portion of any food the first time it is passed offends no one.

But I feel far more disciplined when I do!

In a restaurant, splitting, bagging, leaving offends no one.

But I feel far more disciplined when I do!

Saying a polite "No, thank you ... I'm fully satisfied" when offered a second serving offends no one.

But I feel far more disciplined when I do!

Asking for a smaller sized dessert BEFORE it is served offends no one.

But I feel far more disciplined when I do!

This is especially true now that I have learned to SAVOR each bite of the smaller portion!

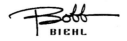
BIEHL

At Your

"IDEAL WEIGHT"

You will not hear

(Or, need to think of yourself as ...)

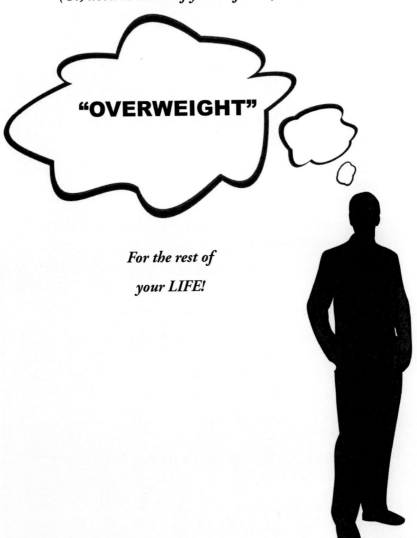

For the rest of

your LIFE!

CHAPTER 7

UNLEARNING
"Clean Up Your Plate"!

FEELING "SATISFIED" — YOU DO NOT HAVE TO "CLEAN UP YOUR PLATE"!

Most of us were raised to think leaving food on our plate is a horrible thing. I agree that being <u>purposefully</u> wasteful is not a good thing, and it is TRULY sad there are actually hungry people starving in this world. BUT being made to feel guilty and intimidated into overeating unwanted food doesn't actually help any of those who are struggling, and is also not going to help us live a long life. This is one "guilt trip" we need to UNLEARN! Eating those last few bites that push you into the realm of STUFFED doesn't affect anyone but YOU.

Before we move on from this idea, let me say if you are still thinking about those less fortunate, channel your passion into helping in some other way, e.g. volunteer at a soup kitchen or donate canned goods, instead of eating MORE in the name of helping others. HELP others in a HEALTHY way!

If you are giving yourself less, and are satisfied before it is gone, that is OKAY. Try packing it in a container to eat later. Even if it is something that will not save, it is not necessary you eat it, to put yourself into stuffed mode. Say it with me: "I DO NOT need to clean my plate! I will STOP when I am SATISFIED!"

quick tip: FROM A HELPFUL READER

Yesterday I was sharing with my daughter and son-in-law about your book. My son-in-law, who is a doctor, had one practical suggestion: To help with portion control was to use a smaller plate! He said his grandparents' plates were/are about the size of our salad plates – they didn't fight the weight problems many of us have.
— R.

quick tip: FROM A HELPFUL READER

When you feel full, put your napkin on your plate and cover what food is left. This helps those of us that were taught to eat everything on our plate not to feel so guilty! ☺ *— P.*

SATISFIED THINKER

"

The reference to "cleaning your plate" is an admonition from our parents / grandparents / teachers since early childhood! Instructing me to "UNLEARN IT" is genius! – L.

"

Thin Thought

*A key to
DROPPING
to my IDEAL
WEIGHT
and STAYING
at my IDEAL
WEIGHT
for LIFE!*

**I ORDER

WHAT-

EVER I

WANT –

THEN

SPLIT IT

/ BAG IT /

LEAVE IT!**

ORDERING WHATEVER YOU WANT IN A RESTAURANT

When was the last time you heard that on a diet? With the THINKING MAN Diet, you really can, because it is a LIFESTYLE change. You will not have to avoid the food you love the most for the rest of your life! You will just have to learn to enjoy it in MODERATION! So keep going to your favorite restaurants! You don't have to stay away from them (because of a short-term diet) for the rest of your life!

If you are eating in a restaurant with a friend(s):

1. Let your first thought be SPLITTING something you both enjoy.

2. Let your second thought be eating ½ of your favorite meal and asking for a "doggy bag", eating the rest as a second meal at home.

3. Let your third thought be just to leave the second ½ on your plate (and have the server toss it)!

Play the "LEAVE SOME" game in a restaurant. When you are served very large portions, at least leave the crust or the edge of a piece of bread, or consider eating the hamburger insides and leaving the bun or a piece of it. Never feel pressured to eat more food just to "clean up your plate"!

In the *THINKING WOMAN DIET* book (written for the women in your life), my granddaughter, Jillian Williams, tells this story:

Every single time I have been pregnant, I have craved things I could not have. My sister has severe peanut allergies, so it was recommended I not ingest peanuts the entire time I was pregnant. Want to guess what my worst craving was? You got it – peanut butter and jelly … with ALL FOUR pregnancies. Trust me, I can tell you a little about being denied what you love! Every time after delivering a baby, peanut butter and jelly sandwiches were what I had in the hospital, truthfully, EVERY meal for days! That mental picture was not for you to imagine me stuffing my face with PB&J, but to remind you that when we are told we CAN'T have something, we CRAVE for it even more.

What we are denied we crave even more!
Go to any restaurant you want and order whatever you want…
then split it, bag it, or leave it!

---

quick tip: FROM A HELPFUL READER

I made it a rule for myself that I would avoid certain things until I reached my goal. I can't tell you how many times I was tempted to order fish and chips in the last 6 months. But for just a few items like that, I told myself, 'As soon as I reach my "IDEAL WEIGHT", I will have that in moderation again.' – W.

> *The concept of eating what you like to eat but less of it makes sense and is very logical."* – F.

Thin Thought

A key to DROPPING to my IDEAL WEIGHT and STAYING at my IDEAL WEIGHT for LIFE!

19

I THINK MORE ABOUT MY "IDEAL WEIGHT" THAN MY "MONEY"!

RESISTING "BUT I PAID FOR IT" THINKING

I was constantly justifying my eating with those types of thoughts, even if I didn't really like what I was putting in my mouth! It is crucial to your success on the THINKING MAN Diet to keep more focused on your "IDEAL WEIGHT" than on the $2 worth of food you might be leaving on your plate.

Just for argument's sake, it is actually far worse for you monetarily to eat those last few bites. If you are gorging, chances are you are gaining more weight than you want. If you continue to gain weight, your clothes will no longer fit you and you will have to buy more.

Or if you continue to gain weight, you might need to go to the doctor more because of your weight causing other issues. Is your co-pay $2? Instead of feeling guilty over those last two bites, be proud of yourself for being able to commit to reaching your "IDEAL

WEIGHT" and staying there!!

Next time you are asked, "Would you like a small, medium, or super large drink?" Don't look at the PRICE! There is a reason advertisers spend BILLIONS on getting you to supersize. It puts more money in their pockets – and more pounds on your body! When you look at the price, it is easy to think it is only a few pennies more, and is so good! We have decided to savor, to eat smaller portions and to really enjoy our food ... and drinks.

Enjoy eating the things you enjoy, but don't fall into the "supersize" trap! I can't wait for you to start following these principles, smiling when you step on the scale in the morning and reaching your "IDEAL WEIGHT".

quick tip: FROM A HELPFUL READER

Trading water (with a lemon) is a great trade off ... also health benefits associated with increased water consumption. – R.

These are habits ... which are invisible to everyone but you. These are habits ... which can help you stay at your "IDEAL WEIGHT" for the rest of your life!

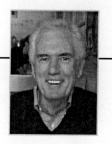

HOW I ACTUALLY FEEL ABOUT: UNLEARNING – "CLEAN UP YOUR PLATE"!

"Leave some" food on my plate in a restaurant has become one of my favorite "secret games". Seeing how much food I have the discipline to leave on my plate once my stomach is satisfied is actually fun! When at home or at a dinner party with friends, I remember to simply take less as the situation allows without offending the host / hostess, always remembering the inviolate rule, "Never offend the cook!"

I honestly no longer enjoy feeling full" or "stuffed" – in fact, I feel miserable. When "full+" I realize I have just gobbled my way to a "stuffed" state. I have added hundreds of calories I really didn't want since I passed the point of "Diminishing Pleasure" many bites back.

I feel zero guilt leaving food on my plate. I would far rather feel bad for leaving food than feel bad for being overweight.

Today, I've actually formed a habit of constantly looking for ways to eat less, which feels great. I'm no longer looking for loopholes to eat more.

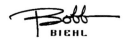

BIEHL

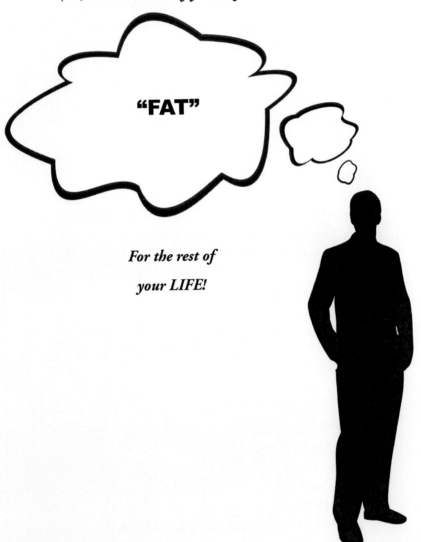

CHAPTER 8

KEEPING
Your New Thinking A <u>Secret!</u>

Thin Thought

*A key to
DROPPING
to my IDEAL
WEIGHT
and STAYING
at my IDEAL
WEIGHT
for LIFE!*

20

**I KEEP

MY

"THINKING

MAN DIET"

A PERSON-

AL SECRET!**

DECIDING IF YOU WANT ANY OF YOUR FRIENDS TO KNOW

Please don't misunderstand – I am not saying you HAVE to keep it a secret or that you absolutely CANNOT tell anyone you are following the THINKING MAN Diet. It would actually be better for me if you told EVERYONE you know to RUN, not walk, and buy the THINKING MAN Diet book for themselves!

However, the THINKING MAN Diet wants you to use the THIN THOUGHTS for yourself, not to impress others. Unless you decide to tell others, each of the THIN THOUGHTS can be totally invisible to your friends!

Hold yourself accountable to reaching your "IDEAL WEIGHT" while eating foods you love, without having to tell a single person!

The last reason to keep the THINKING MAN Diet a secret is PERSONAL satisfaction. It feels great to have other people recognize your weight loss, but remember you are doing it for YOU, not for others to notice. If you keep it a secret and then people do notice, it feels even greater! Your friends and family won't know how you did it, because they haven't seen you change your foods, dietary habits, or exercise program!

Thin Thought

*A key to
DROPPING
to my IDEAL
WEIGHT
and STAYING
at my IDEAL
WEIGHT
for LIFE!*

21

**I CAN
RELAX ...
NO ONE
WATCH-
ES WHAT
I DON'T
EAT!**

SEEING NO ONE WATCHES WHAT
I DON'T EAT!

Your friends watch what you DO EAT!
No one cares what you DO NOT eat!
No one notices (or cares) if an overweight
man says "No, thank you" to a second
piece of pie.

Everyone notices if he says "Yes, please" to
a second piece ... or even a third!

HEARING "YOU HAVE LOST WEIGHT!"

Nothing motivates like results! Having others notice is great! It might take some time for others to notice your weight loss – don't let that discourage you! There will be a time when those around you will take notice – enjoy it! The best part is when you see people you haven't seen in a while looking shocked at your transformation! Once this thought becomes a reality, use it to motivate yourself to stay at your "IDEAL WEIGHT"! Put big changes into practice, grow to the point where these changes are your "NEW NORMAL", and enjoy the fruits of your labor – the satisfaction of KEEPING IT OFF!

SATISFIED THINKER

" *There is not a family I know without a weight issue somewhere ... and it is no secret! — D* "

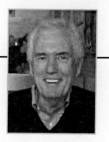

HOW I ACTUALLY FEEL ABOUT:
KEEPING – MY THINKING
A SECRET!

I never wanted to be the butt of family jokes about my weight. I certainly didn't want them hearing I was on a diet! I was afraid they would be watching every single bite I put in my mouth and thinking ... "He has no self-discipline ... no wonder he's so overweight!"

I can't express the great relief I felt when this simple principle hit my brain for the first time: "NO ONE WATCHES WHAT YOU DON'T EAT"! It was like I had been handed another intricate brass key that unlocks the secret of dieting. I didn't have to tell anyone! As a matter of fact, they were so busy gobbling food they wouldn't even notice ... until I had lost a lot of weight! AHA!

An additional pleasure came when I finally realized I was dieting for ME, not for what they would or wouldn't say or what they would or wouldn't do or how much they did or didn't weigh! I was doing it for me! It was MY SECRET!

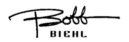

BIEHL

At Your
"IDEAL WEIGHT"

You will not hear

(Or, need to think of yourself as ...)

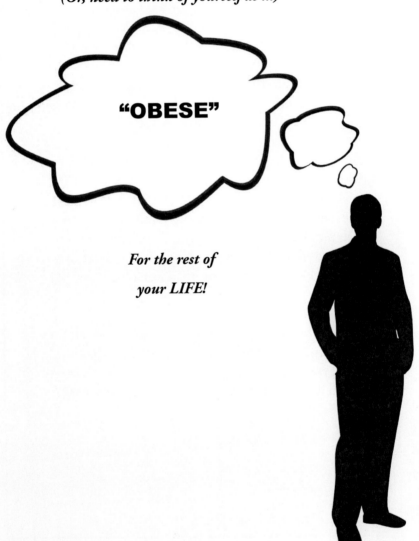

"OBESE"

For the rest of

your LIFE!

CHAPTER 9

WATCHING
Your <u>Self-Image</u> Turn Far More Positive!

Thin Thought

A key to DROPPING to my IDEAL WEIGHT and STAYING at my IDEAL WEIGHT for LIFE!

I'M REDUCING THE PAIN OF HEARING ... "OVERWEIGHT" OR "OBESE"!

USING EMOTIONAL PAIN TO MAKE YOU STRONGER!

Most of the reasons to start the THINKING MAN Diet have already been covered. However, there is one very important reason to start the THINKING MAN Diet we have not covered, and it is ridding yourself of EMOTIONAL pain of hearing (thinking) words like "OVERWEIGHT" or "OBESE"!

If you are reading the *THINKING MAN Diet*, it is because you want to reach your "IDEAL WEIGHT", meaning, you are not CURRENTLY at that weight. If you are like me, you have had weight to lose for a while. I have spent most of my adult life overweight. When you are overweight, or obese, those words are incredibly hurtful. Someone who has never struggled with weight issues can't understand how those words can affect us.

Instead of letting past words hurt you, use them to make you stronger and even more determined to follow your THIN THOUGHTS and see the changes take you towards your "IDEAL WEIGHT" and away from emotional pain! Allow the positive comments from others start replacing the pain you have experienced in the past.

This is so crucial to forming a healthier you, both inside and out. Say it with me!

"REDUCING my emotional pain at words like OVERWEIGHT, FAT, or OBESE feels GREAT!

---

quick tip: FROM A HELPFUL READER

Imagine what it would feel like walking into a party, meeting your wife at a fancy restaurant, dancing with lighter steps, going to your reunion, etc. Imagine how you will feel and dwell on this positive future memory. – B.

SATISFIED THINKER

"*When I was a young man ... I honestly think the first word most of my close friends would have used to describe me would have been ... HANDSOME!*

For the past few years, they look at me and immediately think OVERWEIGHT / FAT.

I really want them to think of me as HANDSOME again! – J."

DEVELOPING A MORE POSITIVE SELF-IMAGE WITH WORDS!

Your self-image is the sum total of all of the WORDS you use to describe yourself!

If you think of yourself as
FAT …
OVERWEIGHT …
UNDISCIPLINED …
UNAPPEALING …
UNHEALTHY …
then you have a NEGATIVE SELF-IMAGE.

As you approach your "IDEAL WEIGHT", your self-image will begin to change. If you think of yourself as …
THIN …
AT YOUR "IDEAL WEIGHT" …
SELF-DISCIPLINED …
SEXY …
HEALTHY …
then you have a far more POSITIVE SELF-IMAGE.

As you approach your "IDEAL WEIGHT", you will be far more positive about your entire self-image!

DEVELOPING — A MORE POSITIVE SELF-IMAGE IN YOUR APPEARANCE!

As you lose weight, give away some of your old baggy clothes to a friend or to a thrift store in your area!

Buy some great new clothes that fit you thinner body! Buying new clothes, and throwing out the old baggy ones, helps improve your self-image! Don't keep 3-4 sizes of clothes clogging up your closet as "backup" like you did with your "Lose 10 pound in 10 days" diets. It's time to "really mean it" with the THINKING MAN Diet.

SATISFIED THINKER

At my former weight, people typically guessed I was over 60. A friend recently told me I look 48! And I feel 38! Thank you! – N.

SATISFIED THINKER

My belt size has gone from a 42 to a 38 and still shrinking. – R.

CELEBRATE!

SATISFIED THINKER

Like you suggested, I thought about it for a minute. What would it actually mean to:
- *My health*   • *My appearance*
- *My sex life*   • *My self-confidence*
- *My self-respect*

if I could get to my "IDEAL WEIGHT" and STAY THERE using the THINKING MAN DIET?

I'M STARTING TODAY! – J.

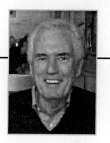

HOW I ACTUALLY FEEL ABOUT:
MY SELF-IMAGE TURNING
MORE POSITIVE

As I began dropping 43 pounds over a period of approximately eight months, my self-image began adjusting a day at a time. My clothes started bagging. My belt literally ran out of holes. What do you think this weight loss did for the way I felt about myself? Believe me, my self-image changed into a more positive view of myself!

I no longer had the hidden fear of one day seeing myself (or friends seeing me) as OBESE, in my later years!

Then came the day when I actually gave 2-3 (new) large black trash bags packed with clothes (some nearly new) to a much larger friend, telling him, "These no longer fit. Take what you want and give the rest to your favorite thrift store!" Then I had a lady who does tailoring re-size 20-30 of my favorite suits, pants, shirts, blazers etc. to save some of the cost of restocking my closet. Did it ever feel great to be able to really fit in smaller clothes!

One of the unexpected negative feelings, which came with losing so much weight was moving from large-sized shirts to medium. At first I struggled a bit with this transition. Somehow it didn't seem as masculine and strong. Then I realized this is exactly what I'd been working toward for the past few months and really enjoyed the new and tailored medium-sized clothes!

One other unexpected side effect: Because I actually lost over 40 pounds, my face began to show more wrinkles. Several months later, my skin has adjusted. Even though I still have plenty of wrinkles at my age, the good news for you is they are not as bad as they were when I first lost the weight. More than a bit vain on my part, but it's another of the unexpected feelings of the THINKING MAN Diet.

Bob
BIEHL

C H A P T E R   1 0

STARTING
Today Step-By-Step Toward Your "Ideal Weight"!

Thin Thought

*A key to
DROPPING
to my IDEAL
WEIGHT
and STAYING
at my IDEAL
WEIGHT
for LIFE!*

**I HAVE
A PROVEN
PLAN TO
DROP TO
/ STAY AT
MY "IDEAL
WEIGHT"!**

STARTING TODAY!

The phrase "Ready, set, GO!" springs to mind, and yet I am not sure it applies. Are you ever really going to feel "ready?" There will always be an excuse, or an event, a reason not to start the process of losing weight. Being even slightly unsure could undermine your readiness. Do not use these excuses! The THINKING MAN Diet is not asking you if you are ready, instead it is asking you if you are DETERMINED. If you have read this book, and agree with its THIN THOUGHTS, just start using them! That isn't nearly as scary as being ready to start (and potentially fail) a new "crash diet."

The THIN THOUGHTS in this book will work for you ... if you follow them! You now have in your hands and mind everything you need to reach your "IDEAL WEIGHT" and stay there for the rest of your life.

" *Love your practical, commonsensical, straightforward approach. – B.* "

To get started:

- ❏ Make very sure you have honestly wrestled with and answered the question "Why?"
- ❏ Set your "IDEAL WEIGHT".
- ❏ Reset your "NEVER-GO-OVER WEIGHT".
- ❏ Take a picture of yourself so you have a baseline and a visual representation of your progress!
- ❏ Weigh every single day ... on a reliable set of scales.
- ❏ Review the THIN THOUGHTS daily until they become lifelong habits.
- ❏ Get EXCITED! You have already started!

" *What is the THINKING MAN DIET worth if it does what it claims? Not sure how to put a price on it. Depending on the person, it could add 10-20 years to his/her life. Not sure you can put a value on that. — P.* "

Thin Thought

*A key to
DROPPING
to my IDEAL
WEIGHT
and STAYING
at my IDEAL
WEIGHT
for LIFE!*

**I AM
BETWEEN
MY
"IDEAL
WEIGHT"
AND MY
"NEVER-
GO-OVER
WEIGHT".**

RESISTING THE TEMPTATION TO QUIT!

Let's face facts: Stopping in the middle of a diet has been a natural temptation in the middle of every diet ... in the history of mankind! Below you will find SUMMARY SHEETS listing the THIN THOUGHTS of the THINKING MAN Diet. Reviewing this list will help you keep resisting the temptation to QUIT! And if you do stop, they can help you get right back on track ASAP!

Carry the SUMMARY SHEET listing the 27 THIN THOUGHTS with you ... whenever you are waiting in a doctor's office, for your car to be serviced, for your children to get out of school. Secretly review each of the 27 THIN THOUGHTS listed below for 100 days, checking each box off on the grid below.

At the end of your first 100 days, you will be able to recite most of the principles without ever trying because you will have them memorized by then. Thinking

THIN THOUGHTS will become your "NEW NORMAL" way of thinking about food and eating. They will come to your memory if you should start getting off track and GRAZING, GOBBLING, OR GORGING!

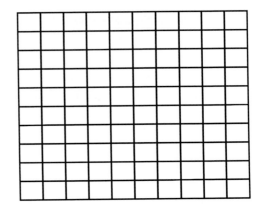

REALITY CHECK:

It's OK to skip a day occasionally … just keep filling in the boxes.
It may actually take you 120 days, which is perfectly OK.
No need to be legalistic. This is just a way to help you brand your "NEW NORMAL" thoughts about food and eating into your brain!

When (not IF) you are tempted to quit, review all of the THIN THOUGHTS … one more time!

---

quick tip: FROM A HELPFUL READER

Work towards a significant reward for reaching your "IDEAL WEIGHT" that will give you lasting pleasure, such as a great bicycle, new elliptical, a new hobby, a new cell phone or acquiring a new painting or sculpture which you can savor and enjoy almost every day. – A.

If you should get discouraged at any time in the next 50+ years, review all 27 of the THIN THOUGHTS!

I have finished the book (actually read most of it twice). Great book. Very practical. I like the emphasis on permanent, achievable life change, not quick-fix, non-sustainable diets. It will be very helpful to me as I continue to my "IDEAL WEIGHT". I'm now 30 pounds closer than I was five months ago. – P.

Thin Thought

A key to
DROPPING
to my IDEAL
WEIGHT
and STAYING
at my IDEAL
WEIGHT
for LIFE!

I WILL

SHARE

THINKING

MAN DIET

WITH

FAMILY

AND

FRIENDS!

HELPING FAMILY AND FRIENDS GET TO THEIR "IDEAL WEIGHT"!

These same THIN THOUGHTS can be very helpful to family and friends when they ask:

How did you DROP TO YOUR IDEAL WEIGHT?

How do you STAY YOUR IDEAL WEIGHT?

" *My wife and I are both following your THIN THOUGHTS and losing weight together. It is a fun project! We help each other. We enjoy "savoring" together. It is fun! — W.* "

Once it has worked for you, please suggest/give the THINKING MAN Diet book to someone else. Help your friends be THINKERS!

www.IDEALWEIGHT4Life.com
www.Facebook.com/IDEALWEIGHT4Life

" *It is good you cared enough to share ... this is life-changing stuff. – D.* "

SUMMARY sheet for the THINKING MAN DIET

KEEP REVIEWING THESE THIN THOUGHTS TO HELP YOU
<u>DROP</u> to YOUR "IDEAL WEIGHT" and
<u>STAY</u> at YOUR "IDEAL WEIGHT" FOR LIFE!

DECIDING your IDEAL WEIGHT.
1. I have set my IDEAL WEIGHT at _____ pounds!
2. I have reset my NEVER GO OVER WEIGHT at _____ pounds.

THINKING for yourself!
3. I really do want to get to my IDEAL WEIGHT because…
4. I will DROP TO MY IDEAL WEIGHT and STAY AT MY IDEAL WEIGHT for ME!
5. I know my current THINKING IS KEEPING ME OVERWEIGHT.

WEIGHING yourself – EVERY morning!
6. I weigh myself NAKED every morning!
7. I weigh myself on a RELIABLE SET OF SCALES!
8. I SLIP … but I get back on "the smiling scales" as soon as possible!
9. I always compare my CURRENT WEIGHT to my IDEAL WEIGHT.

SAVORING every bite!
10. I SAVOR my first bite!
11. I make sure my food tastes great, or I DO NOT EAT IT!
12. I DO NOT
    GRAZE (Eat endlessly)…
    GOBBLE (Eat without thinking)…
    GORGE (Eat after I'm satisfied)!
13. I HATE feeling FULL or STUFFED, so I will stop when I am satisfied.

EATING and DRINKING whatever you want – just <u>LESS</u> of it!

14. I take a moderately sized helping of what I really enjoy eating for my FIRST SERVING!
15. I never take "SECONDS"!
16. I always ask for a smaller dessert, BEFORE it is served!
17. I look for ways to eat less, NOT loopholes to eat more!

UNLEARNING "Clean Up Your Plate"

18. I order whatever I want in a restaurant, and then SPLIT IT / BAG IT / LEAVE IT!
19. I think more about my IDEAL WEIGHT (waist) than my MONEY (waste).

KEEPING your new thinking a <u>secret</u>!

20. I KEEP MY "THINKING WOMAN DIET" ... A PERSONAL SECRET!   (Even from friends)
21. I can relax! No one watches (cares) WHAT I DON'T EAT!
22. I feel great when friends say, "YOU'VE LOST A LOT OF WEIGHT!"

WATCHING your self image turn far more positive!

23. I'm reducing the emotional pain of hearing (OR, THINKNG) words like "OVERWEIGHT" OR "OBESE"!
24. I feel far more positive about myself as I approach my IDEAL WEIGHT!

STARTING today – a step by step plan to your IDEAL WEIGHT!

25. I have a proven step by step plan to TAKE IT OFF! KEEP IT OFF!   (THINKING WOMAN DIET)
26. I have the self–discipline to stay between my IDEAL WEIGHT and my NEVER GO OVER WEIGHT FOR LIFE!
27. I will share these THIN THOUGHTS with my family and friends!

REVIEW: Check off daily for the first 100+ days each time you re-read your 27 THIN THOUGHTS.

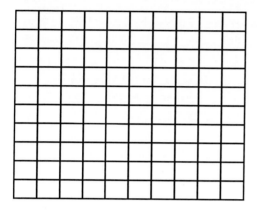

The second possibility for use of this grid is to record your current weight in the top left box. Remember, you are weighing yourself EVERY day. If you keep a record of your weight loss each day, you will see your progress in ink, as well as in the mirror and on your "smiling scales". Look back and realize you did lose last week, even during those hard days. For me, it is so helpful to see my weight coming down. It is up to you how you choose to use the grid, but please use it to help you make progress using the THINKING MAN Diet.

This grid chart is not meant to be legalistic; rather it is to be helpful in making your THIN THOUGHTS your new habits! If you should get DISCOURAGED at any time, review these THIN THOUGHTS to remind yourself of why you committed to this LIFESTYLE change!

REMINDER: THINKING YOUR WAY TO YOUR "IDEAL WEIGHT" – AND STAYING THERE – IS PROFOUNDLY SIMPLE.

Here is the most basic logic of the THINKING MAN Diet: You are:

- Eating what you want to eat ... JUST LESS OF IT!

- Dropping to your "IDEAL WEIGHT".

- Staying under your new "NEVER-GO-OVER WEIGHT".

- Remembering a series of THIN THOUGHTS which becomes your "NEW NORMAL".

- Keeping your new way of thinking about food and eating INVISIBLE TO FRIENDS.

© 2014 – Aylen Publishing – www.IDEALWEIGHT4Life.com

WARNING: Any diet not followed will not work. The THINKING MAN Diet is no exception.

SATISFIED THINKER

" *I have known it had to be a lifestyle commitment and you make that perfectly clear.*
– F. "

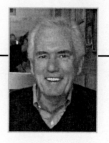

HOW I ACTUALLY FEEL ABOUT: WRAPPING UP THE BOOK!

By now, you may be thinking, "Bobb, you think way too much about food!"

Before I got to my "IDEAL WEIGHT", a high percentage of what I thought about was eating + being overweight! Today, at my "ideal weight", what I think about is savoring and being thin! And I think about helping you:

> Drop to your IDEAL WEIGHT!
> Stay at your IDEAL WEIGHT!

Several men (clients, friends, relatives) I have felt very close to in my life have struggled with the overweight issue. It has hurt me deeply to listen to each talk about:

The pain of being ridiculed by family members, because of being so far overweight.

The embarrassment they have felt at overeating in public, but not knowing how to stop.

The dislike they have for the person staring at them in the mirror because of that person's weight.

Each felt hopelessly trapped in his own belt size. Each had no step-by-step invisible plan he trusted which could make it possible for him to lose the embarrassing weight, let alone have the courage to actually dream about one day getting to his "IDEAL WEIGHT". The idea of "IDEAL WEIGHT", if the idea had occurred to him, would have seemed like an impossible dream.

Today it is not only possible ... but available ... via the THINKING MAN Diet!

REMEMBER:
    I'M NOT A CRASH DIET-IST,
    I'M NOT A DOCTOR,
    I'M NOT A NUTRITIONIST,
    I'M NOT A PHARMACIST,
    I'M NOT A PHYSICAL THERAPIST.

I'm just a person who figured out a combination of profoundly simple THIN THOUGHTS which helped me go in TOTAL SECRET from the most I had ever weighed to my "IDEAL WEIGHT" (TAKE IF OFF!) and keep under my "NEVER-GO-OVER WEIGHT" – with 100% confidence I can "KEEP IT OFF!" for the rest of my life.

Remember, this entire THINKING MAN Diet book is actually just trying to answer two questions:

"Bobb, how did you drop to your IDEAL WEIGHT and stay at your IDEAL WEIGHT?"

"How can I drop to my IDEAL WEIGHT and stay at my IDEAL WEIGHT?"

I sincerely hope you benefit from the THINKING MAN Diet as much as I HAVE ... and STILL DO!

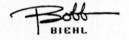
BIEHL

P.S. My trustworthy electronic scales smiled at me this morning ... at 160.4 pounds!